PRAISE FOR *SHOT TO THE HEART*

In January of 2000, I thought I was going in for a cleaning. Surprise, I underwent open heart quintuple bypass surgery instead. From inception to age 70 the human heart beats 2 billion times, at an average of 70 beats per minute. As part of the procedure, I was hooked up to a heart-lung machine ($180 from Amazon) for 42 minutes. That gave me an extra 2940 beats. You do the math!

My emergency surgery is how I met Dr. Karl Krieger. As with many of the people I met that day, Karl has become a lifetime friend. To be clear, Karl is more than a surgeon. Although, dear God, shouldn't that be enough? Karl is a medical savant, miracle worker, genius, magician, and crazy good-looking.

In *Shot to the Heart*, Karl has assembled stories from his life, his practice as a thoracic surgeon, and his time in the O.R. Reading this book you'll understand why I love Dr. Krieger. Thanks for the extra 2940 beats, Karl. We'll be right back.

DAVID LETTERMAN

Dr. Karl Krieger is a surgeon's surgeon. For decades, his gifted hands, stamina, and compassion provided the unsung heart and soul of an illustrious New York City heart surgery program built on catering to the rich and famous. Dr. Krieger has written a stirring memoir that vividly captures the language, the techniques, the flow, and the intensity of open-heart surgery. Dr Krieger makes you feel like you're scrubbed with him in the operating room.

CRAIG R. SMITH, M.D., heart surgeon and author of *Nobility in Small Things*

Karl Hemingway Krieger, a relative of Ernest Hemingway, was in the same creative writing course at Amherst College alongside renowned novelist Scott Turow and historian David Eisenhower. After graduation, he enrolled at the Johns Hopkins School of Medicine, where he was among the few to complete the rigorous program and earn his M.D. in just three years. The Amherst creative writing class ultimately produced three distinguished writers, and this book offers you the opportunity to experience Karl's remarkable writing firsthand.

Shot to the Heart is a true account of his nearly 50-year journey as one of America's most distinguished academic heart surgeons. In it, Karl shares both the disappointments and the rewards of his profession. I know his story is true—because I was there for most of it, spending more hours each day with Karl than with my own family.

O. WAYNE ISOM, MD, Chairman Emeritus, NYP-Weill Cornell Medical College

Karl Krieger, a brilliant cardiac surgeon, takes us with a skilled narrative into the high-stakes world of heart surgery. The reader is invited to follow his early years of preparation and then through the drama of life-saving heart surgery for thousands of patients. He, with other surgeons and operating room attendants we meet, describes how heart surgery extends the lives of children born with coronary abnormalities as well as some of the country's most well-known individuals. *Shot to the Heart* is a unique journey into medicine and the operating room we never expected to take.

FRANK A. BENNACK, JR.
Executive Vice Chairman and former CEO, Hearst Corporation.

SHOT TO THE HEART

Published and distributed by Merack Publishing
Jackson, USA
www.merackpublishing.com

Library of Congress Control Number: 2025900800

Hemingway Krieger, Karl

Shot to the Heart: A Doctor's Stories of Life-Saving Cardiac Surgeries

Author Photo ©John Abbott Photography/New York

ISBN Paperback 978-1-964421-04-9
ISBN Hardcover 978-1-964421-06-3
ISBN eBook 978-1-964421-05-6

SHOT TO THE HEART

A Doctor's Stories of Life-Saving Cardiac Surgeries

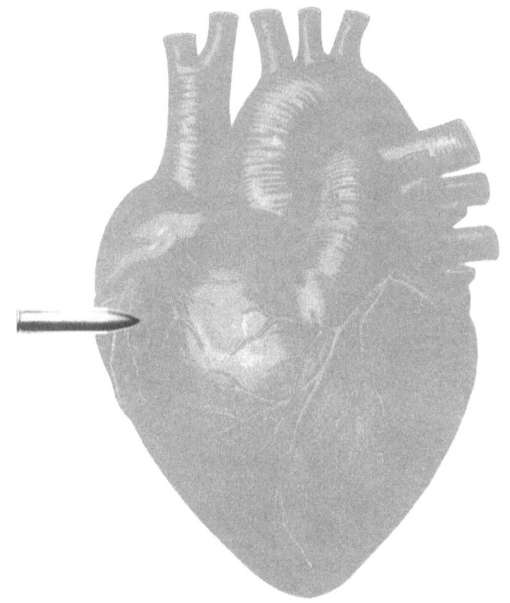

KARL HEMINGWAY KRIEGER, M.D.

CONTENTS

INTRODUCTION

Heart Disease is the most common cause of death in the United States. According to the Centers for Disease Control and Prevention, one American dies every 37 seconds from a cardiovascular event. Cardiac patients can be treated medically most of the time, but the average adult in North America still has a 33% chance of needing a cardiac surgeon during their lifetime.

No one relishes the idea of seeing a cardiothoracic surgeon to discuss their chest being "cracked open." No one looks forward to being connected to a heart-lung machine so that their heart can be cooled to the point it stops beating. And the thought of a surgeon probing around inside your heart to fix a problem that you don't really understand can be quite overwhelming.

So, I have written this book with your questions and well-founded anxieties in mind. I have spent most of my adult life with one or both hands inside someone's chest. I have operated on over 15,000 heart patients in hospitals throughout New York City and the East Coast of the U.S., and I have a good understanding of the problems that lurk beneath the sternal bone.

This book tells stories of real patients, some well-known, who have undergone open-heart surgery. I have fictionalized their names, identifying details, and careproviders to protect their privacy, but the stories are completely true. The stories cover the spectrum of open-heart surgery cases, adult and pediatric, and you are taken through operations, start to finish. Some of the nomenclature will be new, but it should not interfere with your understanding of the story.

Here are first-hand accounts of the problems that surgeons encounter, and insight into their attempts to solve them. You will learn what issues keep surgeons awake at night during the post-operative period.

If you have picked up this book because your internist or cardiologist has recently informed you that heart surgery is in your near future, my sympathies are with you. Yet, when you are told you need heart surgery, you don't want to stick your head in the sand and hope for the best! As a patient, you should know something about the individuals you are trusting with your life, and as much as possible about the harried hospital world you will be a part of.

Welcome. It's time to scrub in.

SHOT TO THE HEART

I was looking forward to helping Phoebe do the takeback. Our coronary artery bypass patient from the morning had bled 1,000ccs of blood into the chest tubes and needed to go back to the operating room for an exploration. Phoebe was a third-year surgical resident, and I liked her. She was smart, she worked hard, and she never complained. She deserved this case, and I wanted to help her get through it.

Cardiac takebacks were perfect teaching cases. Once we opened the sternal incision and drained out the clot that had a chokehold on the heart, the patient always got better. The patient was asleep and had no idea what was going on, but physiologically the brain, kidney, and other organs all welcomed the increased blood flow. The ICU nurses also welcomed the takebacks. They had a two-hour respite while the patient was in the OR, and the patient's family, who had been worried all night about the bleeding, felt relieved. The nurses assured them that the surgeons would stop the bleeding. Everyone felt better after a takeback.

Phoebe and I entered the hospital through the emergency room doors, as usual, and headed for the back elevators to the operating rooms (ORs). It was midnight, and I felt optimistic. The case would only take two hours skin to skin, and we would get some sleep tonight.

Entering the elevator bay, I felt someone grab my arm and say, "Can you help us?" It was the emergency room head nurse who had spotted me. "There is a gunshot wound to the chest coming in . . . cops are bringing him . . . it's a 16-year-old kid . . . they are minutes away . . . can you look at him with us?"

I knew I was the only Cardiothoracic surgeon in the hospital at this time of night, so I said, "Absolutely." I told Phoebe to call the OR and tell the charge nurse to put the "takeback" on hold. I added, "Ask the anesthesiologist in our room to come down to the emergency room STAT. We might need his help."

Within seconds I heard the police siren outside. A police car, sirens blaring, screeched to a stop in the ER loading dock. The orderlies were ready with a mobile stretcher and pulled a body out of the back seat. They loaded the body onto the stretcher and raced to the trauma bay inside the emergency room. The kid was fully grown, maybe 160 pounds, and completely limp and unconscious. There was a circle of blood in the middle of his sweatshirt. I grabbed his wrist and felt a slight pulse. "He's got a pulse." The anesthesiologist from the OR raced into the trauma slot. As calmly as possible, I said, "Tube him, he is not breathing . . . I need a subclavian insertion catheter and a 10cc syringe . . . get his clothes off . . . cut them off . . . I need Ringer's lactate, and I will get blood for stat type and cross . . . I need Epinephrine and bicarbonate and a subclavian line."

Nurses ran in five different directions. They knew their job and had his clothes cut off in seconds. There was a bullet wound in the middle of the sternum, and I knew there was a 90% mortality rate with gunshot wounds to the heart. Yet, this was a kid, and this had to be a low-caliber gunshot from a handgun. I knew we had a "chance."

I grabbed the 10cc syringe and central line catheter. I stuck the left subclavian vein beneath the left clavicle, something I had done a thousand times before. I was suddenly aspirating a full syringe of dark purple blood. I disconnected the syringe, and blood shot out of the end of the catheter as if I had hit the subclavian artery. For two seconds I held my breath; had I hit the artery? No. I was sure of my stick . . . I knew this was venous blood. The central pressure was high, very high. This had to be cardiac tamponade. The bullet had pierced the heart, causing blood to collect and compress the heart, and the heart could barely contract. "Tell the OR he has cardiac tamponade. I will need a sternal saw . . . get a pump in the room, call in a perfusionist . . . STAT. We are on our way up."

The nurse handed me a large-bore IV catheter to thread inside the needle, giving us central access to the venous system. She asked, "What do you want?" I said, "Push in 4 mg of Levophed, 2 amp of bicarb, and a liter of Ringer's lactate.

I asked, "Phoebe, do you still have a pulse?" The answer was "No." I said, "Put a board beneath his back." To the anesthesiologist I asked, "Ted, can you ventilate him okay?" The answer was "Yes."

"Okay, let's get him upstairs . . . someone get the trauma elevator."

There were at least ten nurses and nurses' aides standing around the trauma slot. Gunshot wounds took the highest priority during the night shift, and a gunshot to a kid, especially in the heart, caught everyone's attention.

"Let's get upstairs . . . now!" The ocean of faces parted. We had lost, at most, five minutes in the trauma bay, and every second was critical. I climbed up on the mobile stretcher, straddled the patient, and started pumping on the center of his chest. Phoebe yelled "I got a pulse . . . make way, make way," and we cut through the mass of onlookers.

The elevator ride took thirty seconds. "Phoebe, do you still have a pulse?" "Yes, but only when you pump."

I knew the heart was no longer beating, but we still had a shot at saving him. Each time I pumped on his chest, some oxygenated blood was getting to his brain. With the plate behind his back, the chest was stabilized, and the pumping would be most effective in creating some blood pressure with flow to his brain.

The elevator jolted to a stop. The door opened, and we raced into the operating room. Next to the OR table, I climbed off the stretcher and stopped pumping for thirty seconds as we lifted the body onto the table. I then stood on a six-inch stool and resumed pumping.

I said, "Give all meds through the central line . . . Phoebe, put in a Foley catheter, and give me a big femoral venous line . . . You can cut down if you have to and make it a big volume line . . . Stick in a femoral arterial line for the anesthesia team, and give more Levophed in the central line . . . and more bicarb."

There were twelve people in the room trying to help. We now had a second anesthesiologist, three or four scrub nurses, a medical student, and several surgical residents. All trying to help.

"I am going to keep pumping . . . someone prep his chest with betadine and drape him . . . I need new gloves . . . hook up the Bovie cautery . . . Phoebe, keep working on the femoral lines, then you glove up . . . no time to scrub. Help me open the chest. If we can drain the pericardial space, he should come back . . . he's young."

Three minutes after hitting the operating room, I took a knife and drew a long, deep incision down the middle of his chest. In a normal patient, blood would be squirting in all directions. Because I had stopped pumping, he had no blood pressure and no bleeding. I split open the xiphoid process with a heavy scissor. I then slid my forefinger underneath the sternal bone and over the top of the pericardium. With my left hand I created a space above the sternal notch and dissected downward. I pumped hard on the sternum ten more times and said, "Saw." The scrub nurse, who was a fully trained cardiac surgery regular, handed me a saw that looks like a carpenter's jigsaw. I zipped open the sternum from bottom to top, right down the middle. It took three seconds.

I held out my hand, and the scrub nurse slapped a sternal retractor into my palm. I cranked open the chest cavity about five inches, and I could see the pericardial sack that houses the heart. It was dark purple and tense with blood and clot. "Knife." I cut the pericardium down at the diaphragm, careful not to hit the heart. Suddenly, blood shot up three feet, soaking me and the scrub nurse. It was all venous blood under tension. I opened the sack further, and a liter of dark red blood and clot raced out. I could see the empty heart quivering, no longer able to pump at all. The aorta felt soft. The blood pressure was 30 or less. "Give him more Levophed, more bicarb, and more Ringer's . . . give him blood when you get it . . . I need the paddles . . . do we have a blood gas yet?"

The nurse handed me the internal paddles to shock the heart. "All hands off the table!" "BAM"—the electrical current made the heart jump. Then nothing moved. The heart was still dead. I took my forefinger and flicked the right ventricle. The small amount of current related to the flick was enough to wake up the injured muscle. The heart started a slow, prolonged contraction.

It was painful to watch. The contraction was too slow to pump any blood, but it was no longer fibrillating. I put both my hands in the chest, one on each side of the heart, and compressed both the right and left ventricles, synchronized with each slow contraction. I asked the anesthesiologist to give 2mg of Epinephrine. "He probably needs more bicarb too . . . do we have a blood gas?"

Phoebe had finished lining up the patient. She had catheters in both the arterial and venous circulation, and she was now across the table from me. She said, "I sent a blood gas from the femoral arterial line . . . it will be ready soon." On the monitor a sea of wide wave forms undulated slowly. The heart rhythm was slowly coming back. I kept massaging the ventricles with both hands but less forcibly now. I felt optimistic. The heart had defibrillated with one shock, a good sign it would recover. If the kid's head was okay—that is, if there was no brain damage from low blood flow—then we had a shot at victory.

Over the next half hour, the young man's heart slowly recovered. We were flogging the heart with inotropes. We supported the peripheral circulation with alpha constrictors like Levophed, and we poured in packed red cells and clotting factors to rebuild the blood volume. I could see the bullet's entrance point in the middle of the right ventricle. It was oozing black crankcase dark blood. Lifting the heart gently,

I could see the exit injury in the back wall. The left ventricle, the main pumping chamber of the heart, was left unscathed. This was a critical fact because closing a left ventricular injury was difficult. The right-sided holes were easy to fix. I asked for two pledgeted sutures with 3-0 Prolene. I closed the anterior hole easily.

I then propped the heart up with a moist lap pad so, with Phoebe's help, I could see the posterior exit hole. I placed two stitches so that I could squeeze the hole shut. I didn't sew it closed; I squeezed it closed. From the left side of the table, I asked Phoebe to tie the knot with eight throws. I then lowered the heart carefully back into the pericardial space. The heart had not missed a beat.

Next, I had to locate the bullet. After traversing the sternal bone and both walls of the right ventricle, it had lost steam, and I could feel it buried in the posterior pericardium. I extracted it easily. It was 4mm in diameter and 6mm long, coming from a low-velocity handgun. It had not created much blast damage traversing the sternum and the heart. The posterior mediastinal structures like the esophagus had not been injured. I handed the bullet to Phoebe and said, "This is your first gunshot wound to the heart. I want you to throw the bullet into the metal dish, and I want to hear it clang," as was the tradition with bullets in the operating room. I said to Phoebe, "Welcome to the world of midnight gunshot wounds."

More help was now arriving. A third anesthesiology attending came to look over our patient and help out. The heart was recovering rapidly now. The blood pressure was 90mmHg systolic, and the heart rhythm was nearly normal. The systemic PH had been corrected, and the blood oxygen level was in the normal range. We could see the first trickle of golden juice in the Foley catheter. His kidneys were starting to function.

Phoebe and I traded sides of the table. She was now on the surgeon's side, and I was the first assistant on the left side. It was her job now to stop all the bleeding from the skin down to the sternal bone. Most of the work was done with the electrocautery stopping individual bleeding vessels. It was meticulous, painstaking surgical work. I then helped her place eight steel wires through the sternal bone. These wires, as thick as a pencil lead, would be used to pull the sternum back together and stay in permanently. We put in a substernal chest tube over the heart and individual tubes in both pleural spaces to drain the chest cavities. We did not want blood to collect around the heart or in the pleural spaces. Bleeding would be monitored each hour. We closed the subcutaneous tissue and the skin rapidly, both of us working silently, as fast as possible.

When we transferred the patient to the intensive care unit (ICU) bed, he was perfectly stable. His heart rhythm was normal sinus. Despite the trauma his body had just experienced, his blood pressure was also normal. Phoebe and I and the whole operating room team were elated. We had done our job.

Now the ICU nurses would take over his care. I loved this hospital's group of nurses. They were very experienced and knew their job well. They could be a little harsh with inexperienced house staff, but there was no bullshit. They would keep our patient safe, and if anyone could revive him, it would be this team.

I looked at Phoebe and said, "Good job . . . now we need to take back our coronary bypass patient from today. Remember him? One of the OR nurses told me they have opened up a second operating room for us, and the patient is being transferred down as we speak. I am going to help you get through this case, and we should finish around 5:00 a.m. We will have just enough time to take a shower before starting morning rounds."

At noon the next day, while we were replacing an aortic valve on an 80-year-old, word came from the ICU nurses that our young patient was waking up and moving all extremities. The nurses knew that Phoebe and I would be thrilled. The following day on morning rounds, the patient was fully awake, and we removed his breathing tube. He had minimal bleeding from the three chest tubes, so we removed them in the afternoon. The patient was now talking a mile a minute, seemingly oblivious to his ordeal, and we knew his brain was okay. There was a policeman posted outside his room twenty-four hours a day, and the rumor mill was that the kid was a low-level drug dealer and had been shot by someone in his business. His sister witnessed the shooting from her apartment across the street and immediately called

911. The cops who brought him in had been less than a block away when they got the call. They found him prostrate in the middle of the street, threw him into the back of the cruiser, and raced the three blocks to the ER.

Five days later, the patient was walking around the hospital ward, still talking nonstop like nothing had ever happened. I think his security detail grew tired of his talk, and without asking me or the other doctors they transferred him to the hospital jail. Phoebe and I examined his wound there five days later, and it was healing well. He was then transferred to a jail in lower Manhattan, and we never saw him again.

BITTERROOT

Growing up on a cattle ranch in western Montana, I did not know any doctors. I was never ill, and the only medical person I knew was Dr. Smith, our large animal veterinarian. He was always very friendly to me, and I liked him a lot.

My father was an experienced cattleman, and he took care of most of our veterinary needs. But when we had a serious problem—when a calf was severely lacerated by a barbed wire fence, when a newborn was stuck in the birth canal, or when Buster, our best bull, became so limp he couldn't walk—we called Dr. Smith.

We first telephoned his wife where they lived five miles away and told her our problem. She then contacted him on his truck's short-wave radio, which I thought was very high-tech. He covered a large territory. The Bitterroot Valley was eighty miles long and five miles wide. He would answer the radio, and she would relay our problem. "A bull is down on the K-5 Ranch . . . when can you get there?" He would give us a time, and we would watch for his white medical truck coming from miles away. It was a hospital on wheels. When he arrived, he always seemed to find a solution to our problem. We never had a complex medical situation that he couldn't solve or fix, and I grew up admiring him enormously.

When the time came to apply to college, I assumed I would become a veterinarian too. I had worked hard and done well in all my local high school classes, and my guidance counselor suggested I apply to colleges in the East. He said the colleges were "better in the East" and he thought I would "get in on scholarship." He said the admissions people "like guys from the West." He added, "I have a connection in the Admissions Office at Amherst College in Massachusetts. They might like you."

I applied and got in on a full scholarship, likely due to my tennis achievements. Somehow, despite my rigorous ranch duties, I was able to become Montana's Junior Tennis Champion. It wasn't until I arrived in western Massachusetts that I realized Amherst was an all-boys college. That was my first big shock. The second big surprise occurred when the other students asked about my long-term plans. When I said, "veterinary medicine," I got lots of quizzical and strange looks. Finally, one of my classmates condescendingly said, "You don't go to Amherst College to become an animal doctor, you become a people doctor . . . you take care of humans, not dogs and cats." I did not have a quick reply to that comment. I did not know what to say, and when I inquired at the pre-med office, I was emphatically told, "This is a pre-med office, not a pre-vet program."

I thought about this problem for several months. I knew I was fortunate to have been accepted into Amherst, and I thought maybe the college had a good reason not to want a pre-veterinarian program. I agonized for the whole first semester, and finally, I thought to myself, *I am no longer in the West . . . I am now in the East and have not seen a cow in months. Maybe I should go with the flow. I will think about medical school.* (No intended offense to Dr. Smith.)

Amherst had a killer pre-med program. Over 100 of the 300 first-year students listed themselves as pre-meds. By graduation only 25 remained. I survived not because I was smarter than the others, but because I worked harder. Early in my freshman year, I realized that, coming from a small country high school, I was academically behind 95% of the other freshmen. They typed single-draft English papers answering the question, "What is the real world?" I had no idea where to start with a question like that. In addition, I couldn't type, and typing was mandatory. Every class was a battle for me. Half of my classmates came from prep schools with elite-sounding names like Andover, Exeter, and Choate. There were ten students from one prep school alone, Deerfield, where the headmaster was a prior Amherst graduate.

Fortunately, my "real world" became the Robert Frost Library. Early in my freshman year, I moved into a glass-encased study cubicle on the basement floor, and that cubicle became my home for the next four years. I worked till the library closed at midnight, seven days a week. I had no social life, no freshman drinking parties, and no "road trips" to Smith and Holyoke, the neighboring girls' schools. I was working hard to "catch up" with the other students. I felt I was always behind, and I had to work harder than the others. I was also aware that no matter how hard I worked, studying was easier than working on the ranch. Taking care of livestock in western Montana was a 24/7 occupation. In addition, studying in the library I was always warm and dry. Most of the year in Montana I was cold and wet.

After four years of working hard in the Frost Library, I was ready to apply to medical school. Dr. Hoffman, a genetic biologist who was the pre-med advisor, said, "Montana doesn't have a medical school. Where do you want to go?" and I said, "Where do you recommend?" He replied, "I think you would do well at Johns Hopkins . . . I doubt they have ever had an applicant from Montana. I think they would like you, and you know, 'geographic distribution' might count."

So, I applied to Hopkins, and with Dr. Hoffman's strong recommendation, I was accepted. I bought my first car, an old VW Bug, from a college secretary for $300. I borrowed a used set of license plates and drove at night with all my belongings to Baltimore. An Amherst classmate's mother let me rent a single-room apartment in her home in Fells Point, a short distance from the hospital, for $150 a month. I would live there for the next five years.

For the first two years, the curriculum at Hopkins was a breeze compared to Amherst. Everything we needed to learn was written in a book. To do well on the tests, you had to be willing to study hard, but that was it. There was a massive amount of information to assimilate, but conceptually the work was straightforward.

In the third year of medical school, we started working with patients in a clinical setting. We took histories and did physical exams on real patients, and we made rounds with the house staff on the different hospital services. We learned how to draw blood, start IVs, write orders, and keep notes in the patient's charts. We learned how to talk to patients both in the hospital and in the outpatient clinics. We were learning how to be clinical physicians, and after years of classroom didactics, this new responsibility was welcome.

At night one day a week, I worked an eight-hour shift in the Hopkins Clinical Laboratory doing arterial blood gas measurements, complete blood counts, and urinalysis. I liked the practical nature of the work. When I called an intensive care specialist and reported that a patient's PO_2 was 50mmHg (Low), I felt I was actually participating in patient care, and I liked that feeling. A second blood sample was sent down thirty minutes later and the PO_2 was now 110mmHg (Normal), and I felt I had made a difference. I liked the concept of doing something other than just studying. In the laboratory I felt important.

During Christmas break that year, a crisis struck my family in Montana. While hauling hay on the ranch, my father suffered a major heart attack. He was catheterized and told he needed emergency bypass surgery. This was during the early days of cardiac revascularization, and hospitals in the Northwest were not yet doing bypass surgery. He was flown to Palo Alto, California, and a Stanford surgeon did a necessary triple bypass. I flew in from Baltimore and saw my father the night prior to surgery, and to me, he looked like he would die. My father had been a Marine fighter pilot in World War II, he had played college football at the University of Montana, and he was the strongest man I had ever seen, but now he could barely lift his head off the pillow. Despite his weakness, the surgery went well, and seven days later he was flown back home to Montana.

This whole whirlwind event seemed like a miracle to me, and when I returned to Baltimore, I knew what I wanted to be. I was going into cardiovascular surgery.

That meant after graduating from medical school, I had to complete five years of general surgery training. Then I would need to complete two to three years of cardiac training, and then I hoped to join an academic cardiac surgery practice. That became my plan.

General surgery came first, so on the plane flying back to Baltimore, I started reading Dr. William A. Nolen's bestselling autobiography, *The Making of a Surgeon*. The book detailed his five-year general surgery training program at Bellevue in New York City. Even I knew that Bellevue was one of the largest and best-known city hospitals in the Western world. It was famous because of its massive size and because it was run by the New York University Hospital resident staff. At the time when Nolen wrote his book, residents from Cornell, Columbia, and other metropolitan hospitals had rotated there, but now only NYU doctors staffed the whole hospital.

Bellevue was known as the hospital for the poor, the indigent, the huddling masses of New York City. Anyone who could not afford care at a private hospital was sent to Bellevue. Any homeless person, drug addict, or alcoholic who the NYPD picked up was dropped off at the Bellevue emergency room. Non-English speakers and immigrants new to New York also learned they could seek care at Bellevue.

The attending staff at NYU were told to supervise the patient care at Bellevue, but the daily care orders were written by the NYU resident staff. The surgical residents did 90% of the surgeries, and they took responsibility for patient care, both pre-op and post-op. The medical residents ran the medical services including the emergency room and the outpatient clinics. Bellevue was described as a "resident-run hospital," and that immediately appealed to me.

The training program at Bellevue sounded exciting to me, and it definitely captured my imagination. The residents oversaw the whole hospital and wrote all the orders. It sounded like a great place to train where the residents took all the responsibility.

Johns Hopkins had a more traditional training approach, which had existed for the last 100 years. The chief surgical residents were all relatively old, eight to ten years post-medical school. Most were married and had families, and they seemed old enough to be my father. This was the last year of their formal training, and most would become medical school faculty at schools across the country or take positions in private practice. Senior residents in the hospital were three to four years post-medical school, and they managed the day-to-day activities of the service. They also did the majority of the surgery, always with a Chief Resident or an Attending Surgeon. R1 and R2 residents were at the bottom of the hierarchy. They drew bloods, started IVs, collected lab data, ordered blood cultures, and wrote orders for the nurses. They were the workhorses of the service, and they took their daily orders from all of the more senior residents.

At Hopkins, fourth-year medical students like myself could take a one- to two-month elective rotation on the surgical service to learn how to become surgical interns. The fourth-year student rotated on call every other night with the official surgical intern, and the student intern was directly supervised by a second-year resident. It was the resident's job to teach the sub-intern *all* of the responsibilities of the hospital internship. If the process went well, the medical student might be offered a first-year (or R1) residency position the following year. A surgical internship at Hopkins was one of the most coveted residency positions in the country.

Inspired by Dr. Nolen's book, I applied for and was granted a surgical sub-internship on the "Halstead 4" Service. I worked seven days a week and was on call every other night with an R2 resident as my backup. I was very familiar with the hospital; The R2 resident Dr. Weise and I got along well, and he was a great teacher. Alternating call with me was a Washington, D.C. Medical Center graduate named Alex Jones. He and I did all the dog work, or "scut work" on the service. We drew bloods, started IVs, and collected data that we presented at morning and evening rounds. We also wrote all the orders and did the history and physical exams on new patients. It was a tremendous amount of work, and Alex decided after one month that he had had enough and the work was "too much."

Late one night, he took me aside and said, "I am going to quit." He told the Chief Resident that he would stay until the end of the month. He was then going back to a Boston-based medical center and switching to a different residency. This meant that the Hopkins Surgical Residency Program was one intern short, with nine instead of ten interns. They were in a bind.

William Balmer was the administrative Chief Resident, and he said to the Chief of Surgery, "Our R1 intern is quitting August 1. He is going back to Boston. We are, therefore, down one intern for the whole year. We have a sub-intern who is a fourth-year Hopkins medical student and is on the service now. Is there any way we can keep him for the year? He wants to go into general surgery, followed by cardiac training. He can do the job. He is doing it right now. Otherwise, the surgery department is short an intern for the whole year. What do you think?"

The chief said, "Take him, if he wants the job, but tell him he has to stay two years, not just one. Send him to me, and I'll talk to him. What's his name?"

So, I met the world-famous Chief of Surgery at the famous Johns Hopkins Hospital. He ushered me into his office and said, "I hear you are doing a good job on Halstead 4. I also heard you want to go into surgery, and it seems we have an open slot at the end of the month. William Balmer says you outworked the intern on Halstead 4. When he quits, I can offer you his job, but I must get permission from the Dean of the Medical School because you would skip your whole fourth year of medical school. To make this work for our department, you will need to stay two years, and then I will help you transfer to any program you want in the country. You would go in as a third-year resident. Would this interest you?"

I said, "Absolutely!" and in the back of my mind I was thinking, med school is costing me $10,000 each year and a first-year intern makes about $10,000 a year. This was a $20,000 gain for me. Yet, I would have done it even if I didn't get a penny because I was saving a full year of general surgery training. After my experience with my father, and after reading Nolen's book, I was fixated on cardiac surgery. Taking the job would save me both time and money.

Then the Chief of Surgery asked, "Do you have a locale or program you want to go to as an R3?" I said, "Yes, Sir, I just read William Nolen's book on surgical training, and I would like to work in New York City at the Bellevue–NYU program. Would that be a possibility?" His eyes widened, and he looked at me very seriously. "If you want to go to Bellevue–NYU, the Chief of Surgery is a Hopkins guy. He is one of my closest friends, and he is a great heart surgeon . . . you do a good job for the next two years at Hopkins, and you will have a good shot at securing an R3 position at Bellevue–NYU. This might work out fine."

We shook hands, and I went back to work as a "new" Hopkins surgical intern who was eventually headed to New York City. I had come a long way from the Bitterroot Valley.

LESSONS FROM "THE JOHN"

At major teaching hospitals like NYU, the surgical "on-call" house staff officer was responsible for treating cardiac arrests. At all hours of the day or night, this resident was called for all cardiac catastrophes. It was his or her job to carry an "arrest beeper," and when a patient's heart stopped anywhere in the hospital, or when a heart attack patient's blood pressure dropped precariously low, the beeper would go off. A specific location in the hospital would light up, and he or she would immediately stop doing what they were doing and run to the arrest location.

They would usually arrive at a scene of absolute mayhem. Interns and residents of all different specialties and experiences would be trying to pump on a patient's chest, start IVs and central line catheters, give medications, and hopefully revive the stricken individual. It is the surgeon's responsibility to organize this confusing scene, prioritize the critical care, and keep the patient alive.

As a general surgery resident at NYU hospital, I had considerable experience in this role already. During my first early years of residency, I had done over 100 cardiac arrests on both the medical and surgical services. One memorable Christmas Eve, I supervised seven cardiac arrests over a twelve-hour period. I would run to the bedside, stick an endotracheal tube down the patient's throat, and slide a central line catheter below the collarbone so that intravenous medications could be injected directly into the heart. I would push in appropriate drugs, direct chest compressions, and try to save the patient in any way possible. Despite my efforts, three patients died that night.

The Chief of General Surgery at that hospital, Fred Springer, worked seven days a week, fifty weeks a year. He religiously took the last two weeks off in August to go fishing with his family, but otherwise he was "in the hospital." Even his secretary, Hannah Smith, routinely came in on Sundays. Dr. Springer lectured the house staff, "Patients are just as sick on Sunday as they are on Monday ... don't you forget it."

He ran a very tight ship, and he expected 100% commitment from the surgical house staff. Early on in my third year, when I became aware of his dedication, I mentally took the leap and decided I would be working full time too. I could shower and change my scrubs in the OR locker room, I would sleep wherever possible, usually in empty surgical ICU (SICU) beds, and I scavenged leftover food from the patient's trays. For the next three years, I would visit my apartment across the FDR Drive maybe once a week, usually on Sunday afternoons, mainly to check my mail and pay the bills.

Once I mentally made the commitment to working this hard, my job became easier. There were no competing distractions, no mental anguish about being someplace else. I was "all in," day and night, 24/7.

Halfway through my first year at this teaching hospital, I was rounding on the general surgery service when my beeper went off. I recognized the number as Dr. Springer's office, so I stopped rounds and called immediately. Dr. Springer's assistant picked up the phone on the first ring. She rapidly said, "There is a cardiac arrest in the cath lab, one of FS's [Fred Springer's] patients . . . I cannot find a cardiac fellow or junior attending . . . Springer is scrubbed . . . I think they are all scrubbed . . . I know you are not on the cardiac service, but could you take a look for me?"

When the Boss's office called, there was no debate about priorities. I would never think to say, "Hannah, I am on the general surgery service now, and cardiac is not my responsibility." Instead, I said, "I am on my way." I flew down three flights of stairs to the cath lab, ready for the "worst."

Emile Castro, the Chief of the cath lab, was holding an oxygen mask over the patient's face and he was directing traffic. A cardiology fellow was pounding on the patient's chest, but the arterial line registered a pressure of only

50mmHg. The EKG showed ventricular fibrillation. I said, "Dr. Castro, let me help you ventilate . . . I can tube him." I grabbed an endoscope from the crash cart, gently pushed the doctor away from the patient's head, and quickly stuck a #8 endotracheal tube down the patient's trachea. At this hospital, I had learned to carry endotracheal tubes in my white jacket 24/7. I had the tube securely taped in place within thirty seconds. This guaranteed us a secure airway. I gave the hand bag back to Dr. Castro and said, "Sir, this will make it easier for you to ventilate him."

I went to the left side of the cath lab table and stuck a central line just below the left clavicle. I also carried these catheters and 10cc syringes in my white jacket. Once in place, we could give drugs directly into the heart itself. I asked the cardiology fellow, "How many times have you shocked him? And how much Lidocaine have you given?" He answered, "100mg of Lidocaine and we shocked him four times . . . he didn't convert for even a second." I said, "Give him another 100mg of Lidocaine and some beta blocker through the central line and shock him one more time. I will take over pumping on his chest . . . you must be tired."

The cardioversion, not surprisingly, was not successful, but I now had control of the resuscitation. The fellow had been generating a pressure of 50mmHg, which was woefully inadequate. I slipped into position on the right side of the table, asked the nurse for a small footstool, and started to pump hard. My imaginary goal was to make the sternum touch the spinal column. The blood pressure immediately came up to 100mgHg. At 100mgHg his brain and critical organs would be perfused, and he would have a shot at survival. I said, "We need a Foley catheter passed . . . who can do that?" A nurse timidly raised her hand. I said, "Thank you very much."

While I continued pumping on the patient's chest, I turned my attention back to Dr. Castro. I said, "Do you know the status of the OR cases? Are any cardiac OR rooms available? I doubt we will be able to cardiovert him because of the left main. Maybe the best option is to take him directly into the OR and bypass him. From the pictures I see on your cath screen, it looks like the LAD [left anterior descending] and the circumflex are good targets. It may be our only option. What do you think?"

Dr. Castro said, "I suppose you are right . . . we tried Lidocaine, Pronestyl, and beta blockers with no luck. I don't have any other suggestions." I said, "If we can get him into an OR room, we can cannulate his groin and go on pump. We could cardiovert him, open his chest, and bypass all three coronary arteries. He should come back; he's young."

Suddenly, the patient's right arm, which had been partially secured, lifted up, and the patient took a swing at me. He tried to hit me! With the elevated blood pressure, his brain perfusion was improving, and he was waking up. He was blinking his eyes and trying to shake his head. He probably sensed that someone was pounding on his chest and was hurting him. He was trying to hit back.

I backed off and pumped less hard. The blood pressure dropped to 70mmHg, his arm went limp, and it dropped back down onto the table. I excitedly yelled, "Dr. Castro, His head is okay! He just tried to hit me . . . he's getting enough blood flow to his brain." To the nurse I said, "Please secure his arm so I can get the pressure back up . . . this guy will survive if we can get him to the OR."

Never before had a semi-comatose patient taken a swing at me. This was a very good sign.

Dr. Castro said, "Let me go talk to Dr. Springer and the OR supervisor. I will push them to get us an OR room as soon as possible. I will also talk to the family and get consent for surgery."

The cardiology fellow took Dr. Castro's place at the head of the table and ventilated the patient. I said, "Give him 10mg of morphine so I can pump harder and get his pressure back up." To the nurse I said, "Please send blood for type and cross, get pump bloods for the operating room." I then relaxed for a moment, but I kept the patient's blood pressure over 100mmHg. The cardiology fellow and I were now in a holding pattern.

Twenty minutes had passed when I heard the cath lab door open behind me, and I heard Dr. Springer's voice say, "What are you boys up to? You out rounding up cases for us? What you got here?" He stepped up next to the table, and I said, "Dr. Castro has been looking out for us, sir. This is a fifty-year-old Wall Street executive with a 90% left main and good ventricle. As you can see on the screen, he has three good targets for bypass. We just need to get him to the operating room so you can fix him. He fibrillated when Dr. Castro shot his left main, and we cannot defibrillate him. He has been shocked multiple times. Dr. Castro and his staff have done a great job keeping him alive. In addition, I know his head is okay. Just now he tried to hit me. We just need to get him into OR, sir. How long do you think?"

"Well, they are putting wires in my room and will be out in fifteen minutes . . . then another ten minutes to clean the room. Can you last that long?" I said, "Absolutely, this guy is young . . . this is a good case."

It was a good case because there was an enormous upside to saving this guy. He probably had a family who depended on him. We could do a good job fixing his heart. And he could return to a normal life, with 20-30 years of normalcy. He was not our usual 70- or 80-year-old patient with a poor prognosis. If we got this guy through surgery, he would go from being "dead" to being very much alive, with a very long life ahead of him.

Dr. Springer said, "I am going to talk to the family of the first case. I will then talk to the family of this patient. It will take thirty minutes to clean and sterilize the OR. Jeff Connor will help you with the transfer."

The transfer would be a logistical challenge. We would have to move the patient from the cath lab table to a mobile stretcher. We would then rush down the hall to the operating room and lift him onto the OR table. The whole time

I needed to keep pumping on his chest to maintain some blood pressure.

Jeff Connor was a second-year cardiovascular fellow in his last year of cardiac training, and he was already an accomplished surgeon. He would first assist Dr. Springer during the surgery, and I was hoping they would keep me as a second assistant.

With Jeff's help, the transfer went smoothly. Springer returned to his office and left instructions to call his assistant when we went on bypass. He said, "You may want to go on Fem-Fem bypass to start . . . you guys decide."

Normally, heart surgery is done through a sternotomy incision. The sternum is split down the middle, the pericardial sack around the heart is opened, and the critical heart structures are all right in front of the surgical team. I had always thought of this great exposure as God's gift to cardiac surgeons. We heparinize the patient to prevent blood clotting, and we cannulate the right atrium and the aorta for the bypass run.

It all takes fifteen minutes.

Today, we did not have the luxury of fifteen minutes. I had to keep pumping on the sternum to maintain a blood pressure, so we decided to use an older technique, Fem-Fem bypass. While I kept pumping on the chest, Jeff exposed the left femoral artery and vein. We heparinized the patient and placed cannulas in each structure. We then asked the perfusionist to slowly go on bypass, draining venous blood from the femoral vein cannula. The blood was oxygenated and pumped back into the arterial system via the femoral artery. We were able to flow at three liters/minute, which was adequate to protect his brain.

When I was able to stop pumping on the chest, I raced to the left side of the table, and Jeff took over on the right. He made an incision over the sternum and zipped open the sternal bone, bottom to top, with the sternal saw. We opened the pericardium and cannulated the right atrium with a large venous cannula. We then switched over venous drainage to the right side of the heart. This provided increased blood flow into the pump. We were almost ready to "rock and roll." Jeff said, "Call Springer's assistant to tell the boss we will need him in fifteen minutes."

I had already dropped down to the leg and was dissecting out the left superficial saphenous vein. I would take 35cm from the left side, and Jeff removed 20cm from the right thigh. This would be our conduit or "pipe" to replace the arteries in the heart.

Exactly fifteen minutes later, Dr. Springer entered our room, scrubbed and ready to operate. He was wearing magnifying loops and a headlamp for optimal vision. Most of the coronary vessels were between 1 and 2 mm, and the loops made seeing possible. The suture material we used was as thin as a hair.

Springer replaced Jeff on the right side of the table and said, "Any problems?" Jeff said, "No, sir . . . we haven't looked at the targets, but no problems so far." He switched to my side of the table on the left.

The LAD target was a beautiful 3mm vessel that would help our patient enormously. The circumflex and right arteries were 1½ mm vessels, and they were also relatively good targets. Springer cooled the blood to 28°C. He cut the saphenous vein to appropriate lengths for bypass. He arrested the heart with cold cardioplegia as normal. The three distal anastomoses were done in thirty-five minutes, and Springer released the cross clamp. He then took his time as we rewarmed, and he sewed the proximal anastomosis to the aorta without difficulty.

Springer looked at me and said, "What do you think, doctor? Will he come off bypass without a balloon pump? The targets were pretty good."

I did not know if this was a trick question or not. The balloon pump was a heart support device placed in the femoral artery to help support injured hearts. Springer was known for putting residents and fellows on the spot in our conferences, so I said, "Sir, we were pumping on his chest for two hours pre-op . . . I am sure his heart muscle took a hit; it must be somewhat injured. He is young and will tolerate a balloon pump . . . let Jeff and me stick one in. At M&M (Morbidity and Mortality) conferences you often say, 'safe is better than sorry.'"

He smiled at me and said, "Go ahead. I am going to the office . . . there are patients waiting . . . stick the balloon in, and I am sure you will come off bypass okay. Call me if you have a problem."

He looked at Jeff and said, "Call me when you get to the surgical ICU. It is 4:00 p.m. now; let's make rounds at 6:00 p.m."

He turned to me, "Doctor, thanks for your help. I was told you saved this man's life today. You must have learned a thing or two about cardiac resuscitation while you were down at 'The John.' You know I trained in Baltimore . . . that was my old stomping grounds. I will look forward to having you rotate on the heart service."

Our patient did well. Five days after surgery, I saw him walking in the hallway. Jeff told me that his heart and brain were both okay. There was no evidence of brain damage.

On the eighth day, he was discharged home.

BLACKOUT

I was climbing the stairwell between the third and fourth floors at the hospital one night, where I was a rotating resident, when the lights suddenly went out. I grabbed the railing and continued up but was surprised by my disorientation and the intensity of the darkness. I could not see my own hands. On the fourth-floor landing, I instinctively reached for the doorknob that would open into the intensive care unit.

I pulled open the door, and I expected to see a busy, well-lit, post-operative intensive care unit with nurses sitting in a nursing station, but I was startled to see nothing. Like the stairwell, the ICU was completely black. There were no puffing ventilators, no beeping monitors, no nurses or technical staff, no light of any kind. I said, "Hello . . . hello. It is Dr. Krieger. I am the R3 resident on call tonight. Who is here? What has happened?"

A woman's voice said, "All the lights just went out . . . we have no power. I am looking for our flashlights . . . I know I have flashlights someplace."

I replied, "Is there backup power? This is a hospital . . ."

She answered, "I think so, but I have no idea how to turn it on."

"How many ICU nurses are working tonight?"

"Two. Amanda left a minute ago to go to the bathroom."

"How many patients are on ventilators?"

She answered, "Three," and immediately I thought, *this is not good. This is a real problem . . . three patients with no ventilation and no oxygen.*

I said, "We have to hand ventilate them immediately . . . they are not getting any oxygen . . . where are the flashlights?"

"No flashlight but I have a penlight." I saw a thin beam of light stretch across the room.

I said, "Point out your most ventilator-dependent patient, and I will hand bag him . . . what's your name?"

"Miriam."

She flashed the penlight to my left, and I saw an elderly male struggling to get air. I raced to the bedside, disconnected the non-functioning ventilator, and started hand-bagging the frantic semi-comatose patient. "Miriam, find the flashlights STAT . . . I am okay in the dark. Ask in the hallway for help from the floor nurses. We need someone at the bedside for each ventilated patient . . . grab anyone from the floor."

Miriam disappeared with the penlight into the hallway, and I heard frantic voices from outside. Thirty seconds later, a beam of light from a real flashlight shot across the room, and Miriam and another nurse raced into the unit.

I said, "Just focus on the two non-ventilated patients ... detach the hand bag from the ventilator, attach it to the endotracheal tube, and start ventilating immediately. The patient's CO_2 levels have to be high, so hyperventilate them for 30 seconds, and then hand-ventilate them with 300-400cc tidal volumes. Synchronize their breaths with your breathing, no faster. Each time you take a breath, you give them a breath ... and periodically you check their femoral pulse ... Miriam, how many nurses are on the floor?"

A new voice in the dark answered, "Two."

"So, what's your name?" I asked.

"Edna."

"Well, thank you, Edna, for your help ... how many flashlights are on the floor?"

"We have two more for a total of three, and extra batteries."

"Are you the charge nurse?"

"Yes"

"How many floor patients are there, and how sick are they?"

"We have two pre-ops who are not sick, and six post-ops who are all stable. Most are asleep. We are okay on the floor for now. I just made rounds."

"Great . . . when Amanda finds her way back to the unit, switch places with her . . . then draw up 12mg morphine and give a 4mg IV push to each of the ventilator patients. We want them semi-sedated so they don't buck and fight our ventilation efforts. When that is done, ask one of your floor nurses to take my place, and I want to round on each of the floor patients with you. Some may be frightened without any light or power. Are you okay with that plan?"

"Yes."

Amanda felt her way down the hallway and back into the ICU. I said, "Amanda, please take over Edna's patient and ventilate him. Synchronize each breath with your breathing . . . Edna is going to give all three patients some morphine so they won't struggle and fight the tube. Then, she and I are going to round on the floor patients. I do not see any lights outside the window, and no backup power has come on yet. I think the power failure is not just in the hospital but in the rest of the city too. I hope we will get power soon, but we cannot count on it."

After administering the morphine, it was safer and easier to ventilate the ICU patients. Lily, a floor nurse, came into the unit and took over my patient, and Edna and I took two flashlights onto the floor.

I said, "Let's check blood pressures and pulse rates on all the patients who are awake. We will examine all the IV sites and make sure they have enough fluid hanging to get through the night. We will give urinals to all the males and bedpans to all the females. I don't want anyone trying to find the bathroom in the dark. Let's bring sleeping pills for anyone who wants one and try talking all the patients into taking them. We will tell all the patients that they can yell for help if a problem comes up. The bedside buzzers will not work. They can yell, 'Nurse, I need help.' Either you or I will be within hearing distance all night. I don't want the patients too frightened. Is that okay with you?"

She said, "Yes, Boss."

I wanted to have a game plan in my head on how four nurses and I could get three ICU patients and eight floor patients through the night safely. I thought of Kipling's words:

"If you can keep your head when all about you
Are losing theirs and blaming it on you..."

We had no guarantee the power would come back on any time soon. We all had to "keep our heads." The ICU patients were the big problem. Without functioning ventilators, each patient needed one-on-one nursing support just to breathe. We had no EKG monitoring, no blood pressure documentation, and no mental status checks. All patients had intravenous catheters to provide medication and fluid support. By recording urine output, we had an estimation of cardiac output, but that was all. To make it through the night safely, we needed additional help, and I had no idea where that would come from.

I left Edna with one flashlight to watch the floor patients, and I returned to the ICU. All three patients were doing okay, and I complimented the three nurses on their valiant ventilation efforts. "I know bagging the patients is hard work, but you are doing great. Remember, the natural inclination is to over-ventilate, not under-ventilate, so be careful . . . no faster than your own breathing rate. The floor patients look okay . . . Edna can look after them alone. I will take one flashlight and go look for help."

I hurried down one flight and came out on the third floor, which was a medical floor and not my responsibility. I hoped to find help or an explanation of what had happened. The corridor was completely black, and I made my way with difficulty to the nursing station. Two nurses shone their flashlights on me and one asked, "Are you the cavalry?"

I said, "I wish I were . . . I am general surgery on the fourth floor. We are stable up there for now, but I am looking for help . . . has anyone from security or administration come by?"

They both said, "No."

"Are your patients okay?"

The older nurse said, "So far, but everyone is scared."

I said, "Me too . . . we have three patients on ventilators. They are being hand-bagged, and that is difficult. I am going down to the lobby to look for help . . . or as you say, the 'Cavalry.' Good luck."

I quickly left them and dropped down two flights of stairs into the lobby at the front of the hospital. I had hoped it would be full of nurses and doctors who had rushed into the hospital to help during the blackout crisis. Foolish me. It was empty. Completely empty. No security, no doctors, no emergency personnel . . . and no lights. It was completely black. There was no ambient light from outside coming through the front glass doors. I saw one set of car lights zooming down the street, but nothing more.

"There is no one out there." A gravelly voice came from behind me, and I almost jumped out of my clogs. I spun around and flashed my light in the direction of the voice. An elderly grey-haired janitor was leaning back in his chair with a broom in one hand. I said, "I was looking for help. We need help on the fourth-floor surgical unit . . . Is there anyone around?"

He said, "No doctors or nurses, but I'm around . . . I can help. I can't sweep the floor in the dark, but I can try to help. What can I do?"

I replied, "Thank you very much. My name is Dr. Krieger . . . I'm a surgeon. We need help with the ICU patients. Take my flashlight and I will follow you up the stairs. What's your name?"

"James . . . just call me James."

"James, thank you very much."

I followed James as he slowly climbed the four flights of stairs. He had one hand holding the flashlight and one hand pulling himself up the banister.

On the fourth-floor landing, I waited while James caught his breath. I then pushed open the door into the ICU and led him to the center of the unit. I said, "This is James, he has offered to help us get our ICU patients through the night or until the power returns. I will show him how to hand bag the patients, and he can join the rotation team. This way, you can all have a periodic break. We may be stuck here all night, so James will be a big help. He is generous to offer his assistance. This work is well outside his usual job description."

James quickly learned how to hand-ventilate the patients. In the dark it was mind-numbing work. It was difficult to stay focused, but he was up to the task, and he was soon in a regular rotation with our three experienced nurses.

It was difficult in the dark to evaluate the effectiveness of our ventilation. Without electricity we couldn't rely on machines to help us evaluate the patients. No EKG, no arterial line pressures, no blood gasses. We could feel femoral pulses, we could track the patient's heart rate and take blood pressures, but that was it. So far, all three patients looked stable, but I knew we couldn't continue this forever.

I left the ICU with one flashlight and went out on the floor to check on Edna and the floor patients. She said, "So far, no problems. It has been quiet. No complaints."

I told her about James and said, "He can help like a surgical aide in the ICU. I was lucky to find him." I asked, "Has anyone else come on the floor? Any sign of the cavalry?" She shook her head no.

For the next two hours we were able to maintain the status quo. Edna, our most experienced nurse, constantly rounded on our eight floor patients. She checked vital signs on those awake, and she let the sleeping patients sleep. Except for one spilled bedpan, everyone was doing well.

The ICU was more challenging than the floor. We had no suction to keep the endotracheal tubes clear. Without blood gases we could not gauge if we were over- or under-ventilating the patients. It was hard in the darkness for the nurses and James to stay focused. Edna was periodically giving 2mg of IV morphine to keep the three patients calm. I was constantly checking pulses to guarantee adequate blood pressures. We were able to maintain a urine output of over 50cc an hour on all three patients. That told me we were doing okay.

At 3:00 a.m. I glanced out of the unit door and saw a light at the end of the hallway. It was coming our way. I excitedly proclaimed, "I think there is help on the way!" I opened the ICU door and in stepped Dr. Philip Cooke, Chief of General Surgery. He was the highest-ranked doctor in the hospital. I knew he lived ninety minutes away, so he had driven in the dark all the way to the hospital. He was our only cavalry. He asked, "Are the unit patients all right? . . . has anyone died? . . . do you have enough help with the ventilated patients? . . . what can I do?"

I instantly thought, *of all the attending physicians and house staff associated with this hospital, he was the only doctor who understood the gravity of our situation and had come to help. He was the only physician who came to our rescue.*

Dr. Cooke then confirmed my suspicions of how bad our situation truly was. "There is a widespread blackout in the whole city, a complete blackout. Radio broadcasts say there is looting . . . the situation sounds out of control. How can I help you?"

I said, "Dr. Cooke, thank you for coming. I want you to meet James . . . he laid down his broom to give us a hand, and he was a great help all night. He has been a godsent life-saver for us."

To the janitor I said, "James, take a break, but please don't leave."

With Dr. Cooke's arrival I was able to exhale completely. Some of the pressure I felt all night was suddenly gone. He would share the responsibility with me for whatever happened. Most importantly, with the extra body on our ventilation rotation, James, the nurses, and I could take more breaks. Edna had the floor patients under control, and she had found lukewarm coffee for all of us.

We and our eleven patients would all survive.

Years later, when the rock group The Trammps sang their hit song "The Night the Lights Went Out," I would instinctively flash back to that night like it was yesterday. As a general surgery resident, I spent a harrowing night in the dark on the fourth floor of a city hospital trying to keep three ventilatory-dependent ICU patients alive, and eight surgical patients safe. I was fortunate to have the help of a Chief of General Surgery, four outstanding and skilled nurses, and a brave and hardworking janitor. For all of us, it was a frightening and scary experience.

Fortunately, no one died.

When the power finally came back on the next morning, we all cheered!

THE YORK AVENUE MIRACLE

I loved operating with Dr. Isom. He was an excellent surgeon, he was a gifted and patient teacher, and he liked working with the cardiac surgery fellows. He was also the director of the cardiac training program, so he was officially our boss.

One of his many good ideas was to establish a new position in the Medical Center. He created a third-year general surgery rotation where residents like myself would work into the role of cardiac fellows. These carefully chosen resident doctors would experience an intensive four-month cardiac surgery rotation, with increased patient care responsibility, and our work would also allow the cardiac faculty to evaluate us for possible appointment to the cardiac fellowship three years down the road.

Of all the residents and house staff in the hospital, the cardiac fellows were traditionally considered to be the top of the heap. The majority of fellows were between six to ten years out of medical school, but they officially were still considered to be trainees. Many were already accomplished general surgeons, excellent doctors, and good teachers. When I was a medical student at Johns Hopkins, I held a level of respect for the senior cardiac fellows I worked with similar to that of my own father.

Now I was a third-year general surgery resident, and I felt privileged to have made the cut and be working in this new role of a junior cardiac fellow. I was three weeks into my rotation when Dr. Isom told me I would be assisting him on a complex congenital case the next day. The patient, a six-month-old baby, was born with an AV canal defect and was having trouble breathing. Dr. Isom said the baby was "very sick," the case was a semi-emergency, and we would start the operation early the next morning.

I had heard of babies with AV canal defects, but I had never seen one, and I had never scrubbed in on a very sick baby. That night, I looked up the proposed operation in a book on congenital heart pathology. I read that the surgery was one of the most serious and dangerous operations in all congenital heart surgery. The babies are all born with a malformation of the mitral and tricuspid valves. These valves normally direct blood flow from the atrial chambers of the heart to the right and left ventricles. In this defect, part of the blood flow is in the wrong direction. After birth the babies can tolerate the defect for several months but not much longer. They develop heart failure, and left untreated, most die by the end of the second year.

Usually, corrective surgery is recommended during the first ten months of life, and once repaired, the babies can lead almost normal lives. Our baby, Jessica, was six months old and, like most AV canal infants, was small for her age. On echo she was in borderline heart failure, with a very large left atrium. The left ventricle was also dilated, but it contracted well. Now was the time for Jessica to have her heart repaired. Her mother had been well educated by the pediatric cardiologist on the indications for surgery, and she was eager for us to proceed. She said, "Over the last month Jessica has not been eating well . . . she is losing weight . . . and I am very worried. Please take good care of her . . . we love her to death."

We had been given our marching orders, so that night I made sure the anesthesia, nursing, and OR staff had everything prepared for the next morning.

At 8:00 a.m. the following day, Jessica was given an anesthetic that would keep her asleep pain-free for the next six to eight hours. Dr. Isom strolled into the OR at 8:15 a.m., looking like the conductor of an orchestra. He glanced at me, the pediatric anesthesiologist, and the scrub nurse and said, "Everything ready? Let's rock and roll."

I draped the baby with cloth towels so only her chest was visible. Dr. Isom drew a three-inch incision down the center of her chest and, with a pediatric saw, opened the sternal bone. The arterial blood was relatively dark, consistent with her AV canal diagnosis. We rapidly inserted cannulas into the aorta and both vena cava and went on bypass. The empty heart collapsed to half its baseline size.

We arrested the heart with cold cardioplegia. The right and left atrium were opened, and the mitral and tricuspid valves were carefully examined. I had never seen a congenital case this young, and the cardiac structures seemed very small. Without our magnifying loops and headlamps, I would not have been able to see adequately. Dr. Isom carefully separated the incompetent valve tissue, and he created functional mitral and tricuspid valves. He implanted a Dacron patch, closing the septum between the right and left atrium. He was using a very fine needle and thread, and he placed all interrupted sutures when repairing the valves.

After forty minutes of clamp time, the mitral and tricuspid valve looked relatively normal, and when tested by injecting saline, the leakage or regurgitation was gone. The repair was better than expected. We closed the suture lines in the right and left atrium. We de-aired the heart and slowly restored normal blood flow from the inferior and superior vena cava. The elevated pre-operative pressures in the right and left atrium had returned to normal. The repair looked excellent.

We had cooled the heart muscle to 15°C and the baby's body temperature had dropped to 25°C. It took us forty-five minutes to rewarm safely. We then weaned the baby off the heart-lung machine. We reversed the heparin that had prevented clot formation, and we rapidly closed the sternal incision. We left pediatric chest tubes in the substernal and pleural spaces to drain blood, and we placed a catheter in the atrium to measure the left atrial pressure post-op. This was normal routine, and four hours after the skin incision, we returned Jessica to the pediatric ICU.

I could tell that Dr. Isom felt good about the technical aspects of the surgery, and I smiled as he dramatically told Jessica's mother and father how well he expected Jessica to recover. This was one of the operations where everyone—the OR nurses, the ICU nurses, the surgeons, and the family—all felt good.

"Call for the next case, please."

During the afternoon Dr. Isom and I did a triple coronary artery bypass on a 67-year-old schoolteacher. Technically the distal anastomosis went well, and after cutting the graphs to appropriate lengths, Dr. Isom said, "Trade sides of the table . . . you can sew the proximals to the aorta, can't you?"

"What?" I was shocked at the question. I had not only never sewed a coronary anastomosis, but I had only seen the procedure a couple of times. I hesitated, but only for a moment, because I knew he would guide me through the opportunity, and I quickly switched sides of the table. I overcame my shock, and with his help, the technical part of sewing went well. We weaned the patient off the bypass machine successfully, but all I could think about was that I probably was the only third-year general surgery resident in the United States who had sewed a coronary anastomosis. Thank you, Dr. Isom.

We transferred the bypass patient to the ICU, where he was very stable. When I was confident that he was not bleeding, I hurried upstairs to the pediatric ICU. I wanted to see how Jessica was doing.

Walking into the unit I saw a tall blonde lady who appeared to be in her thirties standing next to Jessica's bed. She was slowly stroking the baby's face. I introduced myself as Dr. Isom's fellow. "I am just checking on Jessica . . . so far, she is doing well. What we worry about the most the night after surgery is bleeding, but so far this has not been a problem." As I spoke, I stripped the tubes running from Jessica's chest to the pediatric pleurovac, and indeed it seemed that the bleeding had stopped. "We will keep her asleep tonight . . . she won't wake up and respond to you until morning, but so far, we're doing great. Do you have any questions?"

She smiled and said, "I am trying to decide if I should stay or go home. I am staying with my sister on York Avenue only a few blocks away and can come back quickly if she starts to wake up . . . I want to be here when she is awake. I don't want her to be frightened."

I answered, "She will most likely sleep all night, but give me your telephone number, and I will call you if she stirs . . . I will be here checking on her most of the night."

Before leaving the pediatric ICU to make evening rounds, I rechecked Jessica's left atrial pressure. When we came out of the operating room it had been 10mmHg, which was in the expected range. I noted it had now risen to 20mmHg. This was higher than I expected but still less than her pre-operative recording. I made a mental note to check it again.

I completed evening rounds on all the cardiac patients—the service was always busy at this hospital—and I didn't return to the pediatric ICU until 8:00 p.m. I noticed that Jessica's mother was still sitting in the ICU waiting room, since parents were not allowed to stay in the pediatric ICU itself. The nurses said she had never left for home, and I slipped unseen into the unit. Jessica looked okay. Her blood pressure was stable, and she was making urine. There was no bleeding, and she was sleeping comfortably. The ICU nurse said, "No problems." I checked the left atrial pressure line and noted the pressure had gone up again into the 25–30mmHg range. That seemed high to me and made me uncomfortable. Time to call Dr. Isom.

I reached him at his home on Long Island, and I said, "The bypass patient is fine, no bleeding. The baby looks okay too. Blood pressure is 110mmHg systolic, she is not bleeding, and she is starting to move a little. My one worry is the LA pressure. Intra-op it was 10–15mmHg after your repair. Initially post-op it was 10–20mmHg, but now it is 25–30mmHg. We have not been giving volume. The Hct is stable. Do we need to worry about it?"

The phone was silent for ten seconds. "Is the mother still around?"

I answered, "Yes." He said, "Well, 25–30 is higher than I would expect, but remember the baby was living at 30–40 pre-op. Let's watch it a few more hours . . . keep me posted." He hung up.

Okay, Isom was the boss and he had all the experience that I didn't have. I found Jessica's mother and said, "Jessica is doing well. One of the pressures inside her heart is higher than expected, but overall, she looks fine. I'm going to be here all night keeping an eye on her . . . you go home, and I will call you if we have a problem." However, Jessica's mother remained vigilant and would not leave the hospital with her daughter in this vulnerable state.

In the adult surgical ICU I could sleep in an unoccupied patient bed, and the nurses would wake me for problems. In the pediatric ICU I had no bed options, so I found a chair meant for a patient's family and sat next to Jessica. I was aware that I didn't know much about post-op pediatric hearts, so I was afraid to leave her, or even think about sleeping.

The baby was stable for the next three hours, but at 2:00 a.m. the blood pressure suddenly dropped to 60mmHg, and the bedside alarm went off. There had been no warning. The pressure had been stable at 100–110mmHg systolic, but now it was 60mmHg, and the baby suddenly looked under-perfused. I flushed the arterial pressure line, but there was no evidence of obstruction. I said to the nurses, "Give her volume, push in 100cc of packed cells, and double her

Epinephrine . . . give her half of a pediatric amp of bicarb and send an arterial blood gas."

All the pediatric nurses in the unit ran to assist, but nothing we did increased the blood pressure. I was very worried, and I gave the head nurse Dr. Isom's phone number and told her to get him on the line. When Isom answered, I told him what had suddenly happened, and what we had done to drive the pressure back up. He was quiet for twenty seconds and then said, "If I speed, it will take me ninety minutes to get to the hospital. The baby will be dead by then. She is probably tamponading from blood around the heart. I'm going to tell you what to do. Get a pencil."

"Number 1: Get a pediatric sternotomy tray from the OR with the pediatric chest retractor . . . tell the OR to include a needle holder and some 5-0 Prolene. Get sterile gloves for you and a nurse to help you."

"Number 2: Prep the chest in the unit with betadine and put sterile drapes around the chest like we did in the OR."

"Number 3: Cut the chest stitches and wires, and open up the chest. Put in the retractor for exposure, and that should make the blood pressure go up if the baby is tamponading."

"Number 4: If the BP is no better, have a second nurse hand-ventilate the baby with 100% oxygen. Then I want you to put purse strings with 5-0 Prolene on the wall of the left atrium, away from the prior suture lines."

"Number 5: Make a cut in the center of the purse string that is big enough for you to pass your finger through. Then stick your finger in the hole, try not to lose any blood, and I want you to stick your finger from the left atrium into the ventricle."

He paused, "Put your finger across into the left ventricular cavity and wiggle it around to dilate the passageway. The blood pressure will disappear with your finger in the valve, so the 'finger fracture' cannot last more than five seconds. Then, pull your finger out and tie the proline suture. If I am right, this is our only chance of saving her." He paused again, and suddenly added, "And one more thing . . . have the pediatric defibrillator ready to shock the heart. She may arrest when your finger is blocking the valve. Good luck. I will be there as soon as possible."

I hung up the phone, and for five seconds I could hardly breathe. These instructions were way above my pay grade. This was not a hernia procedure or a proximal anastomosis. This was pediatric heart surgery. A lot could go wrong. Problems like bleeding, or arrhythmias, or cardiac arrest. I could easily kill this baby with my finger in the heart. And her mother was just outside the door in the waiting room. I had no trained surgical help and no backup. I glanced at the three nurses helping me, and they all had expectant looks on their faces. I said, "Okay, this is what we must do," and told them Dr. Isom's instructions. They still looked at me blankly, incredulously, and they were not moving. I said, "This is our only shot. Otherwise, our baby is dead. I think we can do this . . . we have to do this . . . or the baby has no chance of living. Please, you must help me . . . I cannot do this alone."

The nurses rallied to the call. The help I was asking for was way beyond their duties, but this is why I love ICU nurses. One ran to the OR to get the operating tray. The second started bagging the baby with 100% oxygen, and the head nurse handed me a pair of sterile gloves and prepped the baby with betadine.

Five minutes after I hung up the phone with Dr. Isom, I had draped the baby's chest and had set up a surgical tray on a stand next to the bed. One nurse was passing sterile instruments, and I quickly opened the incision and had the heart exposed. Fortunately, there was no cardiac tamponade and no bleeding around the heart. I then put a purse string suture of 5-0 Prolene in the left atrium. I cut a hole the size of my finger and stuck my right forefinger into the heart chamber. I could actually feel the mitral valve pushing against my fingertip, and I pushed hard into the left ventricle. For three seconds I wiggled my finger to break up and dilate the narrowed mitral valve orifice. I then pulled my finger out and tried the proline suture. I had not lost over 50 ccs of blood in the whole process, and, amazingly, the heart did not arrest or fibrillate. I felt the aorta and sensed that the arterial pressure had increased to at least 70mmHg. The baby was better almost immediately.

I placed betadine-soaked gauze pads over the incision and slowly removed the retractor. The blood pressure was up to 90mmHg now, and the LA pressure was down to 15mmHg. It looked like the procedure had worked. I thanked all the nurses and said, "Someone call the OR and tell them to get a pediatric heart room set up with cardiac anesthesia. We will wait for Dr. Isom and then return the baby to the OR for chest washout and closure. I will talk to her mother in the waiting room and get consent. You were all a great help . . . thank you, thank you. So far, I think we have saved this baby's life. I am so grateful to all of you."

The clock on the wall in the waiting room said 3:00 a.m. The baby's mother was half-asleep, and I woke her up. I told her an abbreviated description of what had just happened with Jessica. I said, "The blood pressure is back to normal now and your baby looks much better. You can come in and see her for a minute . . . it will make you feel better. Dr. Isom is on his way in, and he and I will take Jessica back to the OR for a thorough washout of the chest and closure of her sternum. She is not in pain, and she slept through the whole procedure. I was very worried when the pressure went down, but it is much better now. After we return from the OR, you can come in and sit with her, and then you should go home and get some rest. Come back in the afternoon. We will make sure you are here when she wakes up."

When Dr. Isom got to the hospital, I had Jessica prepped and draped in the OR. He removed the packing from around the heart and irrigated the pericardial space with several liters of warm saline. We measured the pressures in all the cardiac chambers, and the gradient between the left atrium and the left ventricle had disappeared. Most amazing to me was that the mitral valve, despite the rude probing of my forefinger, was not narrowed or leaking. We rapidly closed the chest and returned Jessica to the ICU nurses and her anxious mother.

The remainder of Jessica's post-op course was uneventful. I was able to extubate her in the afternoon of post-op day three, and the drainage tubes were removed on post-op day four. When she was able to sit up in her mother's lap, her mother smiled like the happiest woman in the world. On post-op day eight we allowed Jessica to return home.

Twelve months after that surgery, I was walking home from the hospital one day while it was still light outside, a rare occurrence. I routinely walked on York Avenue to my apartment further downtown. I heard someone yelling my name from a low floor inside an adjacent apartment building. Then a window burst open and I heard, "It is Jessica's mother . . . please wait a minute, and I will bring her down." I turned around and walked back to the doorway and waited. Out walked Jessica's mother with her baby in her arms. "I want you to see my Jessica, doesn't she look wonderful? She's gaining weight, she is starting to stand. Isn't she beautiful? Thank you, thank you, thank you!" Her mother became emotional and started to cry.

It was an emotional moment for me too. I almost felt like crying. Sometimes being a heart surgeon is the greatest job in the whole world, and this was one of those moments.

For the next fifteen years, I saw Jessica and her mother once or twice a year when she was in town visiting her sister. On days when I left the hospital early, I would walk down York Avenue, and Jessica's mother would call my name. I would either go in and visit for a few minutes or she would bring Jessica down to the lobby of their building to show me her beautiful, healthy child.

Over the years, Jessica grew rapidly and was soon almost as tall as her mother. No one except her mother and I would ever know the difficulty she experienced as an infant, and her narrow escape from death. When Jessica was sixteen, the family moved to Virginia, and I never saw them again.

Two years had passed when Jessica's mother sent my office a copy of a college acceptance letter to Princeton. It made me smile.

LOIS'S SISTER

Heart surgeons don't like doing exploratory surgery. When we open a patient's chest, we want to know in advance what we are going to find. With our pre-operative diagnostic studies, we want to have identified the problem with the heart and have a specific plan of how to fix that problem. We don't relish surprises lurking beneath the sternal bone.

During a bypass operation we know pre-operatively what arteries need grafting. The angiogram has told us exactly where the blockages are located. The catheterization has also given us an accurate evaluation of the heart's valve function and the strength of the heart muscle. Combining this information with a medical history and physical exam, we can accurately estimate operative risks within one or two percentage points. We can then confidently share this information with the patient and his or her family. We want to be as straightforward and honest as possible. Heart operations are high risk compared to other types of surgery, and we want the families to be well informed. The worst question you can hear from the family of a patient who is doing poorly after surgery is, "Well, doctor, we never knew the surgery was dangerous; no one told us that . . . he couldn't die, could he?"

The second reason for having a specific game plan before making the incision is that the entire operating team must know their roles in advance. The anesthetic technique and drugs are tailored for each specific patient based on their medical history and on the length of the proposed operation. The assistant surgeons extracting the leg vein during a bypass procedure need to know the exact length of required vein: "I want a left internal mammary dissected for the LAD graft and forty-two centimeters of vein for the two vein grafts." Time is a critical factor in heart surgery and everyone in the operating room must know their exact role and responsibility.

The large majority of heart operations fit this model. That is why I was so uncomfortable with the operation I was about to perform. I was about to make the skin incision on a twenty-three-year-old girl with no diagnosis, no specific operative plan, and no assurance that I could help her at all. It was 10:00 p.m. on a Saturday night, and I was the only heart surgeon in the hospital. I had just finished my residency, and the patient was the sister of one of our ICU nurses. I was nervous and scared, and part of me thought I needed to have my head examined.

I had worked with Lois, our ICU nurse, for five long years of general surgery and cardiac training. I felt we had been through a war together, and I considered her both a friend and a trusted colleague. On Saturday morning rounds, she had stopped me in the ICU and said, "I need your help." She looked very troubled and anxious. Her sister, Sam, had been in a city hospital with severe shortness of breath for the last seven days. During this time her breathing had not improved, and she had developed generalized weakness and could barely walk. She had previously been treated for endocarditis, an infection on her tricuspid heart valve. After six weeks of intravenous antibiotics, she recovered from the infection. Her blood cultures in the city hospital were negative, and the doctors ruled out a recurrent infection. She had been seen by the infectious disease service, the pulmonary doctors, and the cardiology staff. No one knew why she was so weak and short of breath. Multiple echoes of her heart and CT scans of her chest were negative. Her doctors did not know what to do next, so Lois asked me if we could transfer her to our hospital. "She looks like she is about to die, and my parents are frantic."

Of course, I said yes. Hospital doctors feel a special obligation to their own staff and their families. We bent over backward to help them in any way possible. I had no office help on the weekend, so I called the admitting department personally. "This is the sister of one of our ICU nurses . . . I will make an ICU bed available, and you can send for her immediately."

The admitting office said, "Yes sir, we will send an ambulance right now." I then called three consulting services to examine her as soon as she arrived. The pulmonary doctors would evaluate her ability to breathe and opine on her low blood oxygen level. The cardiology service would re-echo her heart, examine her EKG, and comment on her overall heart function. And I asked the infectious disease consultants to reevaluate her history of endocarditis. If the previous doctors had missed something on her physical exam or her history, I was sure our staff would offer new insight into her problems.

She arrived at our ICU at 10:00 a.m., and one look at her told me something was terribly wrong. She looked very weak, and I knew right away she was critically ill. She was pale, cachectic from not eating, and so weak she could barely answer my questions. She admitted to six months of progressive weakness by saying, "I don't have the energy to do anything."

The weekend consulting services jumped into action. Blood cultures were redrawn, but without a history of fever or elevated white blood cell count, recurrent endocarditis was unlikely. The cardiology staff did a portable echo in the ICU but saw no major abnormality except for an enlarged right atrium and moderate tricuspid regurgitation. The lung consult included a normal lung scan and a pristine, clear chest X-ray. All the consult services commented on her low blood gases, but no explanation was offered. We had placed an arterial line in her wrist to monitor her blood oxygen levels and her blood pressure. Most disturbing was that the sequential oxygen levels, despite inhaled oxygen, were not improving. They were actually getting worse. A normal oxygen level was 90 to 100mmHg, and hers was 50 to 60mmHg and dropping each hour. Low oxygen levels in the bloodstream can lead to damage in every organ in the body, including the heart muscle and brain tissue. The brain and nerve tissue are especially sensitive to inadequate oxygenation, and she was on the brink of serious brain damage.

It was now Saturday evening. Lois, who was following her sister's progress, and I were very nervous and uncomfortable. Giving her sister the high concentration of face-masked oxygen was not helping, and the patient was getting confused and combative. I said, "Lois, I don't know what is going on with Sam, but I do know that she is not improving, and I think we need to tube her. Is that okay with you?" She rapidly agreed. I gave Sam a small dose of morphine and inserted an endotracheal tube into her trachea. This would allow us to ventilate her mechanically and increase the concentration of oxygen in her lungs and her bloodstream. Once asleep, her anxiety, fear, and combativeness would disappear, and our ability to oxygenate her blood would improve significantly. This is normal protocol in situations like this, and in 99% of cases, patients improve dramatically.

Not this time. The oxygen level in Sam's blood did not improve, and if anything, it got worse. I called the cardiac anesthesia team to help us evaluate the patient. I was running out of ideas of what to do. Something was drastically wrong, and I was aware that if we could not solve this dilemma, Sam would not survive the night. I told Lois that I didn't know what to do next. "Tell your family that we do not have good news. We still do not know what is wrong, but we are doing everything possible to help save your sister."

I called Dr. Isom, the Chief of Cardiac Surgery who was approximately three hours away at his summer home on Long Island. I explained the situation with Lois's sister and said, "The only option I can think of is to take her to the operating room and put her on the heart-lung machine so we can oxygenate her blood and protect her brain. She is only twenty-three. Maybe I can find a cardiac problem that is fixable related to the valve. Do you have any other ideas?" After thirty seconds of dead silence, the Chief, who knew Lois well, said "You don't have a choice . . . take her to the OR. Good luck . . . keep me posted."

I grabbed the cardiovascular fellow, Eugene Keating, who was on call that night. He had been following the case with me. He had trained in general surgery at a busy city hospital, and he liked midnight crisis management that resulted in operating room cases. I said, "Call the OR and get a cardiac room setup. Call in a Pump Team to manage the heart-lung machine, and be sure Cardiac Anesthesia is aware. I'm going to talk to the family."

Lois and I found her parents in the cardiac family waiting room. They had accompanied Sam in the ambulance from the city hospital and had been waiting anxiously during the day. I introduced myself as Lois's friend and co-worker, and I outlined in general terms the events of the day. I said,

"We are not sure what is wrong with Sam. We have done everything we can for her medically, but she is getting worse, not better. Our only option, as I and the other doctors see it, is to take her to the operating room. There, we can oxygenate her blood with the heart-lung machine and prevent certain brain damage. This is a temporary fix, but I hope in the operating room we can find a more permanent solution. If there is a mechanical problem with her heart, there is a chance we can fix it. If we don't find a problem, she will not survive the night." Her mother burst into tears and said, "But she will be alright, won't she?" I said, "I hope so . . . we are doing everything we can."

I got up and left Lois with her distraught parents. Distraught myself, I went straight to the operating room and changed into scrubs. Eugene had contacted all the members of the cardiac surgery team to book a tentative 10:00 p.m. operation.

I considered the planned operation to be high-risk and highly experimental. The diagnosis was unclear, and this was not the kind of surgery I wanted to be doing on a Saturday night (or on any night). I had not undergone ten years of training to do experimental surgery on a twenty-three-year-old. On the other hand, in my heart, I did not see any other option. Lois's sister would not survive the night with a PO_2 of 30. I had to try something. In the back of my mind, I kept thinking that the problem was related to the endocarditis two years previously. Up until that time, Sam had never had a pulmonary or cardiac problem of any kind.

The operating team consisted of nine people: two anesthesiologists, Eugene Keating, a surgical PA, and myself, and at the table with us was a scrub nurse and her circulator. There were also two cardiac perfusionists to run the heart-lung machine.

Our patient was intubated so we could progress rapidly. She was prepped with betadine tincture and draped so only her chest was exposed. I took a knife and drew a six-inch skin incision down the middle of her sternum. The bleeding, which should have been bright red, was dark purple because of her low blood oxygen level. We stopped the bleeding with electrocautery, and I opened the breastbone with a sternal saw. Underneath, the heart was tense and bulging up against the pericardial sack. I split the pericardium down the middle, and the right atrium suddenly bulged out. Normally the size of a tennis ball, the right atrium was the size of a softball. It was at least twice normal size. The other cardiac chambers appeared to be normal.

I had expected the right atrium to be somewhat enlarged because of the leakage of the tricuspid valve. The endocarditis was the culprit. But I had never experienced a right atrium like this. It was the largest right atrium I had ever seen.

I quickly heparinized the patient and placed an arterial cannula into the ascending aorta. I put venous cannulas in the superior and inferior vena cava. These cannulas would drain blood from the patient to the heart-lung machine. There the blood would be oxygenated, and then pumped back into the patient's circulation via the aortic cannula. I could then isolate the heart from the circulation, allowing a more careful examination of the heart chambers.

The heart-lung machine spun into action, and I arrested the heart with a cold solution of blood and potassium. I could now open each cardiac chamber and examine them in detail. I started with the right atrium, the only abnormal-appearing chamber. Inside, I saw the endocarditis-damaged tricuspid valve. There was no evidence of an active infection, and although it was severely damaged, it looked repairable. Most importantly, I noted a hole the size of my thumb between the right and left atrium. In normal hearts, there is often a small hole the size of a pencil lead at this location, but this hole was massive, and I suddenly realized what had gone wrong with this young woman's heart. The endocarditis caused the tricuspid valve to leak. This caused the pressure in the right atrium to rise dramatically. The increased pressure over time caused the wall of the right atrium to stretch and enlarge. This also caused the small hole, called the foramen ovale, to enlarge and stretch open. Blood from the high-pressure right atrium was flowing across the hole to the left side of the heart. This blood flow bypassed the lungs completely. Because the flow had not passed through the lungs, it was not oxygenated, and that explained her hypoxia or low blood oxygen levels. When we intubated the patient and used positive pressure to improve her oxygenation, the positive pressure paradoxically had the opposite effect. It made her situation worse. Her already low PO_2 dropped even lower.

My feeling of gloom suddenly disappeared because this was a fixable problem. All I had to do was repair the tricuspid valve to stop the regurgitation or leakage. I then sewed the hole between the right and left atrium closed and directed all the right-sided blood flow into the lungs as in a normal heart. There the blood would be fully oxygenated.

The remainder of the operation was straightforward. I placed a prosthetic ring around the tricuspid valve and repaired the valve leaflets. The ring would prevent dilatation and leakage in the future. I plicated the right atrial wall, making the chamber a more normal size. This part of the operation went rapidly. We removed air from all of the cardiac chambers and reestablished normal blood flow. We rewarmed her body and were able to wean her off the bypass machine without difficulty. The oxygen level in her circulation improved dramatically. Her oxygen levels, which had been 30 to 40mmHg, were now over 200mmHg.

At 1:00 a.m., we returned to the intensive care unit with a very stable and well-oxygenated young lady! Lois and I were thrilled to inform her parents that Sam had survived the surgery and would recover completely. We had found a problem in her heart that had not been diagnosed before the surgery, and it had been repairable. We expected an excellent recovery. It was all good news!

Six months after the surgery, Lois told me that her sister was doing great and had completely recovered from the surgery. She had a new job, a new boyfriend, and a new apartment. Her family was ecstatic with her progress. A year later, Lois said Sam had married her boyfriend, and the couple was expecting their first child. I thought, *Great! You go, girl.* I felt that Lois, her sister, and I had dodged a bullet, and I was thrilled for their new family.

A second year had passed when Lois asked if Sam and her husband could visit me in my office. I thought, *Oh no . . . what is wrong now?* I immediately imagined the worst scenario. She probably had a poorly healed sternal incision or wanted a scar revision. I was not sure what to expect, and Lois refused to tell me the new problem.

Sam and her husband came to my office at the end of office hours and I was surprised to see how healthy and happy she appeared. She was a new person, and I barely recognized her. She said she was doing very well and she had a surprise for me. She rolled a stroller into the office, and she unveiled a beautiful baby boy. "I want to introduce you to our son. He is a great little guy, he almost never cries, and we love him to death.

We named him after our favorite heart surgeon . . . Say hello to your namesake!"

MIRACLE MAN

I loved being a member of my tennis club. Having played competitive tennis since childhood, I played college tennis and worked summers as a teaching professional in Massachusetts for five years. Medical school and postgraduate training in New York City put a halt to my tennis. For twelve years I had not picked up a racquet, so an opportunity to play tennis regularly with a large membership of ex-professional players who now lived and worked in New York seemed like nirvana to me!

I also used the exercise room regularly. The club membership was elderly—few members had ever seen the exercise room, and I enjoyed the privacy of my own "workout space." It was there that Jeff Woodworth, one of the senior club members, found me.

He was almost apologetic when he said, "Sorry to bother you, doctor, but one of the players in our game is down on the court. He doesn't look very good . . . I don't think he is breathing. Can you look at him?"

Jeff was always a gentleman about everything. I knew he would not be asking if he wasn't very worried. I said, "Absolutely," and followed him to the court.

As we entered the tennis facility, I could see a motionless body in tennis clothes near the center of the net. Five or six senior club members, some who I recognized, were standing well off the court, all staring silently at the downed tennis player, and then at me. I walked to the net and grabbed the fallen player's wrist while I rolled him onto his back. His eyes were half closed, glazed over, with pupils dilated and staring straight ahead. Not getting a wrist pulse, I instinctively felt for his femoral artery in his groin. Still no pulse, and he made no attempt at breathing.

This was not a good situation. This approximately seventy-year-old man looked dead. He was not breathing, and he did not respond to stimuli. He was not moving, and he had no pulse. Usually, I recognize "dead" accurately, and he looked very "dead" to me.

The head tennis pro rushed to my side, and I said, "Call 911 . . . tell them there is a cardiac arrest . . . try to get an ambulance team to the nearest hospital, then come back." To Jeff Woodworth I said, "Bring a chair and elevate his legs up onto it." I then thumped the left side of the tennis player's chest with my balled-up fist as hard as I could. One of the bystanders gasped.

There was still no pulse, so I started pumping on his chest. After running hundreds of cardiac arrests in a hospital setting, I have learned how to pump hard. I know what it takes to empty a fibrillating or arrested left ventricle, and the gentle compressions one sees in the movies are useless. The heart sits between the sternum and the spinal column, and I try to squeeze those structures as close together as possible with each pump.

In a hospital ward there is always help available in an arrest situation. One person pumps, and a second person ventilates the patient with a face mask and an Ambu Bag. If we can quickly place an endotracheal tube into the patient's trachea to guarantee direct ventilation, that is optimal. On the tennis court we did not have any way to ventilate this man, and we had no oxygen. I could pump all day, but without some ventilation, I would never get him back. I knew what I had to do next. Mouth-to-mouth resuscitation was the only option.

After ten fast and furious pumps on the chest, I reached up and extended the man's head back, placed my lips over his lips sealing his mouth, squeezed his nose shut with my left hand, and forced my biggest breath into his mouth, and hopefully down into his lungs. I did this three times and then went back to pumping on his chest. Ten hard chest pumps followed by three more of my deepest breaths.

The situation still did not look good. When I first got to the patient, he looked dead—no pulse, no respiration, his skin color a dusky grey, and no spontaneous movement. By all normal criteria, he was dead. I thought there was no chance of saving him. Without the EMS I had no help, no equipment, and no oxygen. To myself I thought, *I will keep working on him for ten more minutes and then declare him "dead."* The members gathered around the court would support my declaration. They would tell everyone we had "done our best." The player "had a cardiac arrest, and he could not be resuscitated."

More than ten minutes passed, and I was about to stop pumping when I noticed that something strange was happening. His skin, which had been a dusky grey, was starting to turn a dusky pink. At first, I could hardly believe my eyes. I was shocked. I thought, *Oh my God, something was working.* Only blood flow with oxygenated blood would change his skin color. If his skin was being oxygenated, so was his brain and heart and all his other critical organs. Suddenly, for the first time, I realized that I actually had a chance at saving this poor guy.

Now I pumped even harder, and I was more forceful about my mouth-to-mouth resuscitation. Between breaths I yelled at the head pro. "Where is EMS? They should be here by now. Call again . . . tell them to hurry." I went back to mouth-to-mouth. Ten hard pumps, three huge breaths.

I was really energized now. I completely forgot about the audience that had now doubled in size. We had a legitimate shot at saving this guy, but I needed the paramedics. We needed to shock his heart with a defibrillator, and we needed to intubate him to guarantee adequate ventilation. I kept pumping even harder, and I kept blowing air into his lungs. Three big breaths, ten hard pumps on the chest.

I was starting to tire when the head pro ran back onto the court. "The stretcher got stuck in the elevator . . . the paramedics are here, but the stretcher is too big for the elevator. They are carrying the equipment down the stairs . . . they are on their way." I thought, *old building, small elevators.* I kept pumping as hard as I could, and I could feel broken ribs on the left side of his chest. This can happen if you are using adequate enough force to revive a patient. I kept blowing air into his lungs as hard as I could. Three big breaths, ten hard pumps.

Within minutes two paramedics ran onto the court. I recognized both from my time in city hospitals. I said, "He has no pulse . . . he must be fibrillating . . . we need to shock him now and then intubate him. Do you have oxygen?"

They nodded yes. They set up the defibrillator, put on the EKG leads, held the pads to his chest, and *BAM!* The tennis player's whole body jumped, but one shock was enough. On the monitor he came back with a heart rhythm. It was an ugly, irregular rhythm, but it looked compatible with life. I grabbed his wrist and could feel a faint pulse. He was still not breathing, so we held a tight face mask over his nose and mouth and ventilated him as best as possible. More equipment arrived, and I placed an endotracheal tube without difficulty. He was easy to ventilate, and within two minutes his skin color was completely pink. I stuck an intravenous line into his arm for fluids and cardiac medication. Things were looking up.

Tennis club employees had freed up the stretcher from the elevator and raced down six flights of narrow stairs to the tennis court. We loaded the patient onto the stretcher for the long trek upstairs. I said, "I'm riding with him to the hospital." Although he had a pulse and a systolic blood pressure of 80, I was still worried about our resuscitation effort and his semi-stable condition. He could rearrest at any moment. He had been down on the court for several minutes before I was summoned.

I pounded on his chest and blew into his lungs for at least fifteen minutes before EMS arrived. I knew that statistically only 5% of patients who arrest out of the hospital will be discharged from the hospital at their baseline mental status. In metropolitan hospitals with ambulance services and state-of-the-art emergency rooms, only 50% of field arrests will survive to get into the hospital. Of the 50% who make it to the hospital, only 10% will leave the hospital without permanent brain damage. Our patient had a 1 in 20 chance of surviving this episode with his brain completely intact.

With the aid of the tennis club's employees, we carried our patient up six flights of stairs to the street level without any mishaps. His heart rhythm was semi-stable, with a palpable pulse, and he was easy to ventilate. The paramedics and I climbed aboard the back of the ambulance, and with sirens blaring, we raced to the hospital. I kept my hand on the radial artery the whole way, and we stopped at the emergency room dock on the river side of the hospital. Rushing through the double doors of the emergency room, I felt a great sigh of relief. We had gone from a situation of having very little help to a location where we had all the best help in the world. The trauma team took over his care . . . and my own pulse, which had been sky high, was sliding down to the normal range.

An arterial line was placed in his wrist for online blood pressure recording. Arterial blood gases were sent STAT so we could evaluate his respiratory status and his blood pH and oxygen levels. A central line IV catheter allowed us to measure his central venous pressure and provide intravenous access for medication directly into his heart. A large volume line allowed us to give additional fluids. A chest X-ray was done within sixty seconds of his arrival, and continuous EKG recording allowed us to stabilize his heart rhythm. Within twenty minutes of arrival, he had a stable heart rate. There was no evidence of ischemic heart damage on the EKG, and he had a supra-normal blood oxygen level. The single heart shock at the tennis club had turned his life around. He now had a sustainable heart rhythm compatible with an ongoing life, and we soon nicknamed him our "Miracle Man."

It took two days for the patient to wake up and regain a normal neurological state. I knew he was going to be okay when he asked me when he could finish his tennis match with his tennis club friends. He had no idea of the crisis he had survived. After extensive studies, the cardiology service diagnosed a cardiomyopathy, and they placed a cardiac defibrillator to prevent a recurrent event. Seven days after admission he returned home, and he was soon able to resume 80% of his normal business activities. Our patient was Philip H Geier Jr., one of the most prominent members of the global advertising community and an ardent philanthropist. He was a legend in the industry, and nothing would hold him back.

Despite our efforts to control the heart's rhythm with the internal defibrillator, over the next twelve months our patient continued to experience chronic arrhythmias of the left ventricle. He required frequent medical hospital admissions, and one and a half years after his first arrest, a heart transplant was recommended. He thought about this recommendation carefully and, with a charming sense of humor, said, "As a lifelong political conservative, you must guarantee the heart comes from a Republican donor." He had a successful heart transplant at the hospital's sister institution uptown. Again, he recovered from the surgery quickly. He resumed his normal business, philanthropic, and political activities. He returned to playing tennis, and I was privileged to play with him at the tennis club multiple times. Over the years, our patient made a substantial gift to each of the two hospitals where he was treated. He became our "Miracle Man" in more than one sense.

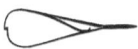

THE FIRST NONAGENARIAN

Dr. Sam Costa bought us dinner at midnight seven nights a week. He would say, "You have to eat something," and he would order Chinese or pizza or hamburgers for delivery to the Cardiac ICU. The cardiac fellows and the nurses on the midnight to 8:00 a.m. shift would congregate at one end of the ICU and gulp down as much food as possible. Often, the cardiac fellows had been scrubbed all day, and Sam's dinner was their only meal. We appreciated the food enormously, and it helped compensate for Sam's constant harassment and yelling during the day. He was the Chairman's go-to attending, and as the Associate Director of the Training Program, he considered it his responsibility to mold us into heart surgeons. He gave us our marching orders daily, orders meant to teach us how to provide premier cardiac care. "Stick a balloon pump in Mrs. Ericson ... then get the

CABG patient opened up, and the internal mammary artery down. The Boss is scrubbing in thirty minutes . . . you better be ready!"

The two-year cardiac training program was the culmination of seven to ten years of surgical training. Soon we would be on our own, and Sam was adamant that we be the best-trained and the busiest surgeons in the country. I was six months from finishing when he said, "Now Doctor, remember this . . . do not operate on anyone over the age of seventy for the first five years in practice . . . 30% will die on you even if you do a perfect operation. If you have a 30% mortality, the cardiologists will stop sending patients to you. Remember, for patients over seventy, the national mortality rate is 30%."

He was trying to help and protect me, but when I became an attending on staff, the only patients referred to me were patients over seventy. The senior attendings, including Costa, took all the younger, lower-risk patients. No one wanted to operate on the seventy-year-old patients, so I became the "Surgeon of the Elderly" by default. I was not happy about it, but I had no other options. In the beginning I tried to select only "good" seventy-year-olds for surgery. I did their bypass and valve operations, and the majority of them did better than expected. Surprisingly, after two years as an attending surgeon, my mortality was less than 5%, not 30%, and I liked working with this patient population. I thought about them as I thought about my own grandmother. She had taught me to read in the second grade, and I was forever grateful. I was fond of this elderly group, as I was fond of her, and over time they became my favorite patients.

After I had worked five years on the surgical faculty, Dr. Isom was named as the new Chief of the cardiovascular service at a nearby city hospital. He offered me a job, saying that it was a move "uptown." He said, "Come and you can operate on anyone you want . . . age is not a limiting factor." I took the offer and was soon doing bypasses, valves, and aortic aneurysms on patients in their seventies and eighties. Working together with the cardiologists, the anesthesia team, and the ICU nurses, we learned how to get these elderly patients through surgery safely. We collected data on octogenarians and heart surgery in which we reported on 100 consecutive bypass patients over eighty years old with a 2.8% mortality on elective cases—truly outstanding results. One of the lessons we learned was that we could not always strive for technical perfection with this elderly group. Striving for perfection was often counterproductive, at times even dangerous. We learned that our primary goal should be to make each patient better, not perfect.

Honestly, I was shocked at how well the patients did. After the paper was published, we were deluged with octogenarians from all over the country, and I grew very fond of this "special" group. I admired their willingness to let me cut open their chests, put them on a heart-lung machine, and try to fix their hearts. I admired and respected their bravery.

One day, a ninety-two-year-old woman from New Jersey called my office. She said she had been turned down for bypass surgery at eight hospitals in New Jersey, Staten Island, and New York City. "They all told me I was too old for heart surgery." She was having daily chest pain; would I see her? Her cardiologist told her I was the "Surgeon of Last Resort."

She came to my office limping because of a chronic childhood injury. She had a very weak heart and blockages of all three coronary arteries. She was not a good operative candidate. I said, "Any surgery on you is very high risk, maybe 50%. You are ninety-two, why would you want to take a 50% risk of not surviving the surgery?"

She raised her head, looked me straight in the eye, and said, "Because of the Yankees."

She was quiet after that, so I said, "What do the Yankees have to do with your heart?"

She replied, "I have been a Yankee fan all of my life. I have been to games in all three Yankee Stadiums. I saw Babe Ruth play in his first game as a Yankee. I saw all the great Yankee players: Ruth, Gehrig, DiMaggio, Mantle, and Maris. The Yankees have not won a World Series in the last eleven years, and I think that this year's Yankee team (the year was 1998) is the greatest Yankee team ever." With tears in her eyes she continued, "I would like to see them win one more World Series before I die."

As a lifelong Yankee fan myself, I said to my staff, "Sign her up . . . she is a baseball lover." I understood this woman's passion and her thinking, and her answer was good enough for me. I called the patient's daughter, who confirmed her mother's feelings. "She has some chest pain daily, but she lives for the Yankees. She thinks they can win this year, and she doesn't want to miss the event."

The next week, we did the operation, a triple bypass, and the patient did great. With the increased blood supply, the heart muscle got stronger. The heart's ability to eject blood went from an ejection fraction of 20% to an ejection fraction of 40%. At 20% her life expectancy would be measured in months. At 40% she could live for years. She had no complications from the surgery, and her angina disappeared. Seven days after the surgery, she was discharged to her daughter's home.

That summer, she was able to attend many Yankee games, and Yankee fans will remember that the Yankees did indeed win the 1998 World Series.

A member of my office staff called Steinbrenner's office in Yankee Stadium and told his staff about our "special patient." The Yankee office responded with free Yankee tickets, hats, jackets, and other paraphernalia for the patient and her family. She was offered an opportunity to throw out an "opening pitch," which she declined. I don't think she felt strong enough to throw a baseball the required sixty feet.

The patient continued to do well for several years. The Yankees did equally well, and she saw the Yankees win a total of three consecutive World Series, 1998, 1999, and 2000.

A year later, at age ninety-six, she passed away from a non-cardiac-related illness. Her daughter called to inform me about her passing and to say that on behalf of the family, she wanted to thank me and the staff at the hospital. She said, "The last four years of her life were some of the best years of her life."

How could I not like and appreciate this patient? I admired her strength and bravery. I admired her love of the Yankees. I admired her family support, and I see her as a representative for all the ultra-elderly that our medical society too often neglects and pushes aside just because of their age.

Her success became a game-changer for ninety-year-olds with heart disease. Many medical centers across the country now consider nonagenarian candidates for open-heart surgery.

"SOME CHICKEN SHIT HOSPITAL"

As the most junior attending on the cardiac surgery staff, I was the surgeon who was called in the dead of night for hospital emergencies. Most of the attending surgeons lived in Westchester with their families, and it was a trek for them to rush to the hospital in the middle of the night.

The ICU staff and the emergency room doctors had developed a habit of calling me for the late-night problems, even if I was not the official attending responsible for the patient. I lived a few blocks away and could be at the bedside in minutes. At this time, I had no wife and no children, and I never made the hospital staff feel bad about calling me with a problem.

In anticipation of the late-night phone calls, I made it a habit of checking the ICU and the emergency room before leaving the hospital. In the ICU I would find the night-shift charge nurse and say, "Miranda, is everything okay? Are you going to need me tonight, or is there anything you want me to look at before I go home?" Most times, all was quiet, and I would grab the elevator down to the ER. There, I would find the attending in charge and say, "Dr. Schiller, is there anything I need to know before I get out of here?" Usually he said, "Go home . . . we have one fresh myocardial infarction (MI), but that is it . . . see you tomorrow."

The routine worked well for everyone, especially me. There was nothing worse than trudging home, taking a shower, getting into bed, and having the phone ring . . . just as I was falling asleep.

Holidays could be very busy on the heart service, so I made it a routine not to check out until well after midnight. One New Year's Eve, I walked into the ER, which looked surprisingly quiet, and I saw Dr. Schiller sitting comfortably in front of a bank of monitors. "Hey, Pete, you are looking very relaxed for New Year's Eve . . . do you have anything I should be interested in?" He smiled and said, "Quiet so far . . ." And then he hesitated. "Well, there is one patient you might find interesting . . . about an hour ago we admitted a neurosurgeon from Minnesota. He is in town on the way to the Caribbean, and he is staying at The Plaza. He had some chest and back pain, and he called 911. The ambulance was there in minutes. He told the EMT techs, 'I have a real problem . . . don't take me to some chicken shit hospital . . . take me someplace good.' So, the driver dropped him here . . . he is a rule-out MI. His EKG looks okay and his cardiac enzymes are negative so far. He is a little hypotensive, so I'm giving him some fluid. You might take a look at him and tell me what you think. His chest X-ray is on the screen in his cubicle."

One of the ER nurses walked me back to the cubicle, and I saw a white male in his late sixties who looked agitated and uncomfortable. I introduced myself and said, "Doctor, what bothers you the most?" He said, "My back is killing me . . . I didn't do anything to hurt my back . . . I had some suitcases . . . that's it. But it is killing me . . . and it's a pulsatile pain . . . it throbs." I did not like the sound of that. A myocardial infarction can manifest as back pain, but it is almost never a throbbing pain. I listened to his chest. His heart sounds were soft, his heart rate was less than 60, no murmurs. The chest X-ray looked normal.

I went back to Pete and said, "I'm not sure he has a primary cardiac problem. His back pain worries me, and he looks sick. If his enzymes stay negative, can you get a chest CT scan tonight? I do not like his looks." Pete suddenly looked alarmed. "Are you thinking a dissection?"

I nodded yes.

"Well, a CT scan poses a challenge, but I think we can do it. We will have to call in a tech to get it done. We do not have a scanner in the ER . . . he will have to be taken upstairs . . . and it will be a hassle on New Year's Eve night."

I said, "It is worth the hassle . . . I don't like his looks . . . I am going up to my office to stick around. Can you call me when it's done?"

A dissection occurs when the inner layer of the aorta, the intima, tears spontaneously, and blood leaks into the wall of the aorta. When this happens, most patients experience a tearing sensation in the chest. Other patients present with less severe pain, and their symptoms mimic those of an acute heart attack. The leaking blood can create a false channel between the layers of the aorta . . . or the aorta may rupture completely, leading to sudden death. What worried me most about the neurosurgeon was the pulsatile nature of his pain. This sounded to me more like a dissection than a heart attack.

A CT scan of the chest was usually diagnostic, but it would be hard to schedule on New Year's Eve. The hospital had just initiated a new 24/7 CT service, and I knew Dr. Schiller would do everything possible to get the test done. Waiting for the usual morning staff could be dangerous.

I took the elevator to our offices on the twentieth floor. I didn't expect anyone to be there, but, most importantly, I had a couch, pillow, and blanket waiting for me. On nights like this, I could quickly go to sleep knowing that there was a telephone six inches from my head on the coffee table in front of me. As backup, I had my beeper in my white jacket. Schiller had two ways of reaching me, and he knew I was only two minutes by elevator from the ER.

The call came at 2:30 a.m. I picked up the ringing phone and all I heard was, "He's got it . . . the dissection is all the way down to the diaphragm." I immediately said, "Pete, can you call the cath lab and get the on-call cardiologist to do an emergency cath? I need to know the status of his coronary arteries and the aortic valve . . . I am on my way down."

Before I ran for the elevator, I paged Stuart Smith, the cardiovascular fellow on my team. "Stuart, we have a dissection brewing in the ER. We will have to do it tonight. Call cardiac anesthesia and the pump team, and notify the OR staff. Tell them I want to make the skin incision in two hours at 5:00 a.m. The patient is a doctor."

I took the back elevator down to the emergency room floor, hurried to the ER, and found Pete talking to the patient in his cubicle. He was preparing him for the cardiac cath procedure. "We need to inject dye to evaluate the status of your coronary arteries. We will also evaluate the valves inside your heart and calculate the strength of the heart muscle. The surgical team needs this information to complete the aortic repair safely."

The patient was listening intently despite his obvious back discomfort. I said, "Is your back pain getting worse, or is it better than two hours ago?" He said, "It is about the same, but it is the worst pain I have ever experienced. Are you sure it is a dissection?"

Pete answered, "The radiologist is 95% sure . . . your ascending aorta is twice the normal size. It has to be fixed before it ruptures completely. The only other thing it could be is a rupturing aortic aneurysm, but either way, it has to be fixed in the operating room tonight. Your pain sounds more like a dissection."

He said, "Okay . . . can you call my daughter? She's also a physician . . . I will give you her number."

The daughter did not sound shocked when I woke her at her home in Staten Island. "He has been having some chest pain over the last year, and his blood pressure runs high. He doesn't like his internist, and I don't think he takes his blood pressure pills. If he has coronary blockages, what will you do?"

I replied, "We will fix everything that we can fix safely. He will be cathed before going to the OR. We will not finish the surgery before 8:00 or 9:00 a.m. How can I reach you?"

"I am getting dressed now . . . I can be there in two hours," she replied.

I said, "His operative risk is in the 10–20% range. There is a 2–5% risk of neurological injury . . . but if we don't operate, I don't think he will survive the night."

After a pause she answered, "Good luck."

I always felt comfortable operating on doctors or their families. Being in the medical profession, they had knowledge of the pathophysiology of the disease process and the risks of the surgery. I did not have to sugarcoat the problems that could occur in the operating room or postoperatively. I felt I could always just stick to the facts.

The cath confirmed the aortic dissection, and it demonstrated a 90% blockage in the LAD—the most important coronary artery in the heart. It would require a bypass. The good news was that the aortic valve was not leaking, and the left ventricle was in good shape, with the ejection fraction normal. All we had to do was replace the ascending aorta before it ruptured completely and do a bypass to the blocked LAD artery.

The operating team would consist of myself and cardiac fellow, Dr. Smith, who was in the last year of his fellowship training. We had a third-year medical student who had just rotated on our service. He could have gone home over the holiday, but he said he wanted to "stick around because he liked the action" on our service. There was a cardiac anesthesiologist attending and his fellow, two perfusionists to run the heart-lung machine, a scrub nurse to pass instruments, and a circulating nurse who did everything else.

At 5:00 a.m. exactly I made a skin incision in the left groin and dissected out the femoral artery and vein. I would eventually use the artery as the inflow cannulation site for the heart-lung machine. I then made a long incision directly over the length of the sternal bone and right in the midline. I quickly used a cautery to stop most of the skin and subcutaneous bleeding. I then carefully created a plane beneath the sternal bone with my forefinger. I could feel the dissected aorta pulsating against the back of my finger. I zipped open the sternum with a sternal saw. Underneath the pericardium I could see the bluish, distended, pulsating aorta. Carefully, I opened the pericardial sack, letting the bloody pericardial fluid rush out. There was no frank bleeding because the outer adventitial layer of the aorta remained intact.

I said to the anesthesiologist, "Give heparin." The anesthesia team injected the blood thinner that had been drawn up into syringes. Now I had to move fast before the aorta ruptured completely. I quickly put cannulation sutures in the right atrium. I dropped back to the groin and made a transverse incision in the femoral artery. I stuck a 20 French cannula inside and sutured it to the skin tissue. I quickly shoved a #50 Bardex venous cannula into the right atrium. "Go on bypass." The heart-lung machine spun into action.

Once on bypass, I felt safe. The heart was beating, but it was no longer pumping blood. All the venous blood was directed into the "pump," not the heart. It was oxygenated and then redirected into the rest of the body via the femoral artery. There was no longer a risk that the dissected aorta would rupture.

I now had time to dissect the internal mammary artery off the inside of the left chest wall. This would be used as conduit to bypass the obstructed LAD coronary artery.

My next goal was to arrest the heart completely. I cooled the systemic blood to 25°C and cross-clamped the aorta at the base of the arch vessels. I opened the dissected aorta, revealing the lumen of the aorta and the two separated layers of the aortic wall. I injected a solution of blood and potassium that would cool the heart muscle and stop it from beating. I packed the surface of the heart with ice slush. With the heart muscle at 10°C, I would have sixty minutes to replace the ascending aorta and complete the bypass to the LAD.

Replacing the aorta was one of the most critical steps in the surgery. I sewed one end of the Dacron graft to the aortic wall just above the coronary ostia. The distal anastomosis was more difficult. The dissected aorta was fragile, and I had to support it with Teflon felt. I then anastomosed the mammary artery to the LAD. This was the most straightforward part of the operation. I removed the air from inside the heart and the Dacron graft. I gradually opened the cross clamp on the aorta, being very careful to prevent air from entering the systemic circulation.

Over the next hour, we gradually rewarmed the systemic blood and the whole body. The core temperature had dropped to 25°C, which had protected all the organs in the body, especially the brain.

Once the body temperature reached 36°C, we weaned the patient off the bypass machine. With a return to normal circulation, we needed to evaluate the heart muscle to rule out cardiac muscle damage during the period of cardiac arrest. With the increased coronary blood flow down the LAD graft, the patient bounced off bypass with completely normal heart function. Kidney function had remained normal during the whole operation, and we would not evaluate brain function until the patient was awake. I did not expect a problem. Technically, the operation had gone well.

Protamine was given to reverse the anticoagulation effect of the heparin. Over the next hour, we meticulously cauterized all the bleeding sites related to the surgery. Bleedings from the suture lines were oversewn and treated with topical anticoagulants. This was the part of the operation where the operative team could exhale, and tension in the room was less palpable. Everyone paid attention to their jobs:

the surgeons had to close the chest, the anesthesia team had to monitor the patient's cardiac function and vital signs, and the circulating nurse was on the phone with the Cardiac ICU preparing the nurses for our arrival. We all had our jobs to do, but our anxiety about the fate of our patient had melted away.

Transferring the patient to the Cardiac ICU was uneventful. A fresh team of nurses and ICU doctors swarmed the patient and took over his care. They cleaned and covered his incisions with dressings, they monitored his vital signs, and they kept me posted on the bleeding from the tubes we had inserted into his chest and mediastinum. I could walk away from the bedside confident he would receive the best ICU care in the world.

I found the doctor's daughter in the family waiting room and described the operation and reviewed our post-operative plans with her. Being a doctor, she was very knowledgeable about the procedure, and she asked few questions.

Within twenty-four hours, our patient was extubated and talking. His heart remained strong, and the chest tubes were removed forty-eight hours after the surgery. By post-op day three, he was walking in the hallway, and on post-op day seven, his daughter took him to her home on Staten Island to recover. A month later, he returned to work full-time in Minnesota, and for ten consecutive years, he sent me a card on New Year's Day telling me about his activities and accomplishments.

Soon after our patient's discharge from the hospital, Dr. Schiller and I scheduled a meeting with the hospital CEO.

We told him the story of our neurosurgeon with an aortic dissection, initially diagnosed as a myocardial infarction. "It is almost impossible to get a CT scan on a holiday or weekend night! We need a CT scanner in the ER, a technician to run it, and a radiologist available to read it . . . it should take us only twenty minutes to scan the whole body."

Six months later, our emergency room CT scanner was up and running.

TAKING CARE OF EMILY

I cross-clamped the aorta of the first bypass patient of the day and said, "Start the cardioplegia at 200 . . . and bring up the ice slush. What is the injection pressure?"

When no one answered, I glanced up to the head of the table. Above the drapes I expected to see Emily Wilson, one of our cardiac nurses and one of my closest friends in the hospital. She should have been looking down at the open chest, watching the heart arrest with me. No one was there.

I rotated closer to the drapes so I could see the whole area above the OR table, and I saw Emily crumpled into a ball, leaning back on her stool. "Emily—are you alright?"

She looked pale and distressed. She mumbled, "I've got some kind of chest pain . . . I don't feel right."

I thought *Uh oh, this is not good.* Emily was not a complainer! We had the heart arrested, and one of our nurses did not feel good and looked bad. It was obvious that Emily was in trouble, and if she was in trouble, we were all in trouble. This was a four-alarm fire. As calm as possible, I said to the circulating nurse, "Barbara, get Ron Spencer in here . . . STAT. Get a wheelchair, and I want Ron (who was the anesthesia fellow on the case) to take Emily to the emergency room. Then, go into the nursing office and tell the secretary we need another cardiac nurse in here ASAP."

Normally, we could not proceed without a full team in the room, but temporarily I thought we would be safe. The heart had arrested, and it would take me thirty minutes to complete the distal anastomoses of our patient, a fifty-five-year-old high school teacher. Then, I could remove the cross clamp, and the heart would be re-perfused. During the next thirty minutes we would warm the patient, and I would sew in the proximal anastomoses. It would be a full hour before I absolutely had to have an anesthesiologist in the room.

Ron Spencer ran into the room. I said, "Ron, get a wheelchair for Emily . . . she is having chest pain. Take her down the back elevators, straight into the emergency room . . . tell the ER attending who Emily is and that she may be having an acute MI. No matter what the doctor says, insist that she get an EKG and enzymes . . ."

"And Ron, one more thing, pretend Emily is the President of the United States . . . do not let her out of your sight. If she fibrillates, shock her . . . and keep me posted. Also, call the Chief of Cardiac Surgery and let him know what is happening."

Ron had a wheelchair in seconds and with the help of the circulating nurse, lifted Emily from the stool into the chair. He would have her in the ER within minutes, and her diagnostic workup would get started.

I refocused on the heart in front of me. It had arrested from the cardioplegia, and I could start sewing on the bypass grafts. I said to the heart-lung machine perfusionist, "Without Emily, you and I will have to manage the blood pressure ... keep it 50mmHg and stay cold ... I will use a lot of slush."

Thankfully, the coronary anastomoses went well. We had good targets for the bypass grafts. Our conduits taken from the legs and the chest wall were excellent. After finishing all the anastomoses, we weaned the patient off the heart-lung machine, and the patient's heart resumed pumping blood with ease. The heart muscle was enjoying more blood supply than it had experienced in years. I could usually tell in the operating room which patients would do well post-op by how well they weaned off the "pump" (the heart-lung machine). Most of the time, cardiac bypass surgery was very rewarding for the patient, the patient's family, and all the involved physicians. Usually everyone came out a winner.

When the patient rolled out of the operating room headed for the post-op ICU, I raced down the back stairs to the emergency room. I spotted Ron near one of the exam rooms and asked, "How is she?"

He answered, "Her vital signs are stable, but her enzymes are coming back positive. She is in sinus tach with some ST segment changes in the anterior leads. They are doing an echo right now. The EF is down slightly, but it is not bad. She is still having some pain, but it got better when we started nitroglycerin."

"Have you notified the cath lab?"

"Not yet."

I said, "I am going to run upstairs and talk to Brown . . . he is in charge this week. She needs to be cathed ASAP . . . she might have a left main. Do not let her out of your sight!"

I took the elevator to the cath lab. I found Gerry Brown, who was the Chief of the catheterization laboratory. I said, "Emily Wilson from the nursing department is in the ER right now. She is having chest pain with positive enzymes . . . her EF is okay. When can you cath her? She may be a candidate for an angioplasty, or she may need an IAPB (intra-aortic balloon pump) and a bypass . . . when do you want her?"

He replied, "We are coming out of Lab 4 right now . . . we can take her as soon as the room is clean . . . I'd say twenty minutes. Give me her full name and history number . . . I will send a fellow down to get her ready."

I called my office and asked for my Nurse Practitioner. I said, "Call the family from the first case and tell them that everything went well. They can see him in the post-op ICU at 2:00 p.m. Most importantly, Emily Wilson is in the ER with chest pain. She is spilling enzymes. Brown is getting ready to cath her in the next hour. She may need surgery . . . call Emily's husband and let him know that he should come to the hospital. Then go to the ER and have a look at Emily yourself. Ron Spencer is with her. Try to make her feel comfortable, and keep me posted."

I didn't want anything bad to happen to Emily. She was a critical member of the cardiac surgery team, and I liked her a lot. When I first came to the hospital, she was genuinely nice to me; unlike many of the staff who resented the arrival of a new heart surgeon, she welcomed me. She consistently went out of her way to help me and make me feel at home. She was old enough to be my mother, and she treated me like an adopted son. I was not going to let anything bad happen to Emily Wilson.

The second bypass operation that day went as smoothly as the first. The patient, a seventy-five-year-old retired fireman, had good target vessels, and we had good bypass conduit. The heart was strong, and we completed the surgery in three hours, skin to skin.

I called the Nurse Practitioner from the operating room for an update on Emily Wilson. She said that Dr. Brown had finished the cath, and Emily had an 80% left main lesion with triple vessel disease. He had placed an intra-aortic balloon pump to support her heart. "He says she will need bypass surgery ASAP. She is not a candidate for angioplasty, but she has three good target vessels for bypass. With IABP support and IV nitroglycerin, her angina has disappeared, and she is resting comfortably in the CCU (cardiac care unit)."

I responded to my Nurse Practitioner, "Thanks, good work. Put her on the OR schedule for first case in the morning. Ask her husband to stay at the bedside, and I will be up to talk to them in thirty minutes. You can call the family on today's second case and tell them everything went well . . . they can see him about an hour from now in the post-op ICU. Then you go home. We will have a big day tomorrow."

Before seeing Emily and her husband, I needed to review her films. The cath lab made a visual recording, a 30mm film, of the cath procedure for the cardiology and surgical staff. We studied the films in detail to see if we could create a detour for blood flow to the heart muscle. If one considered the coronary arteries as pipes carrying blood to the heart muscle, and if those pipes were clogged with plaque, it was the surgeon's job to create a detour for the blood to flow around the blockages. The new pipe or conduit were veins recovered from the patient's legs and an artery, the internal mammary artery (IMA), dissected down from the chest wall.

It all sounds complicated, but the goal is straightforward: the cardiovascular surgeon installs new pipes to replace the old blocked pipes. It's as simple as that.

All three of the main arteries in Emily's heart had severe proximal blockages. With this knowledge I made a diagram for Emily and her husband. I explained how we would remove the vein from her legs to use as conduit for two of the bypasses, and I added that for the LAD vessel on the front of her heart, we would use the IMA from the chest wall as conduit. Emily had an intimate understanding of our plan, and her husband nodded his agreement. "Emily will be going into the OR at 7:00 a.m., so you will want to come early, Mr. Wilson. She will sleep the entire day, and the Nurse Practitioner from my office will keep you posted on our progress. The chances of her coming through well are greater than 90%. The worst complication is a 1% risk of a stroke. Without the surgery she will not leave the hospital."

I ran up the stairs to the surgical ICU. I had to check the two post-ops from today and make sure there was no excess bleeding from the chest tubes. The cardiac fellows would keep track of the patients all night and would call me if any problems developed. I was not too worried because the cases had both technically gone well.

I was more worried about Emily. Her coronary blockages were severe. Fortunately, the intra-aortic balloon pump was supporting her coronary blood flow and assisting with some of the work of the heart.

At home, I told my wife, "I feel like I am operating on my own mother in the morning." Before going to bed, I received two late-night telephone calls, one from the Chief of the Anesthesia Department and one from the CEO of the hospital. They reminded me that Emily had been at the hospital for over thirty-five years. "She is one of our best nurses at our medical center, and we are all very concerned about her welfare."

I arrived at the hospital early the next morning. I wanted to make rounds with the residents to check the post-op patients, but most importantly, I wanted to be in the operating room when the anesthesia team put Emily to sleep. Normally, I would not come into the OR until the chest was opened by the fellow, but I was nervous with Emily. Because of her anatomy, she could have a fatal arrhythmia at any time, and she would be hard to resuscitate.

Fortunately, she tolerated the induction of anesthesia with a stable blood pressure. We opened the chest cavity and dissected the left IMA from the chest wall. We planned to sew it to the LAD vessel on the front of the heart because the LAD was the most important and the largest target. We recovered the saphenous veins from the thighs for the other bypasses. I put cannulas into her aorta and the right atrium. We started the heart-lung machine, which would allow us to arrest or stop her heart from beating. Then, we planned to sew the grafts onto the tiny 1.5mm coronary arteries.

The cardiac arrest went smoothly. We cooled the pump blood to 25°C and injected her heart muscle with cardioplegia at 10°C. I added a topical slush solution to further cool the heart muscle. In this cooled state, the heart metabolism almost stopped completely, and I had thirty minutes to sew my grafts to the coronary arteries.

The first two anastomoses to the right coronary artery and the circumflex went well. The targets were excellent, but when I checked the blood flow in Emily's internal mammary artery graft, I was shocked at its poor flow. My assistant described it best, "She has a little old lady mammary; we cannot use that thing." He was right, and I quickly harvested more vein to use for the all-important LAD graft. This was a significant setback because the LAD target in Emily's heart was her best target, and without the IMA we would be using a less-than-optimal conduit. Long-term patency of the IMA graft at ten years was greater than 90%; vein graft patency was significantly less.

The remainder of the operation was uneventful. We weaned Emily off the heart-lung machine easily. Her EKG looked good, and her heart function was normal. She had not sustained any permanent damage to the heart. All three grafts were functioning well, and flow measurements were excellent. Even the LAD graft had excellent flow. We closed the chest quickly with eight sternal wires. Bleeding was minimal, and I insisted on a subcuticular plastic closure technique. I wanted Emily to be proud of her skin incision.

Emily's post-op course was benign. She was walking on post-op day two, and she spent only five days total in the hospital. Thirty days after discharge, she returned to work. I encouraged her to take three months of accumulated vacation time, but she insisted on an early return. She was adamant that she felt well, and she wanted to keep an "eye" on me.

Emily worked a routine cardiac nursing schedule for the next five years, and she only retired when she reached the mandatory retirement age of 75. She took up traveling and visited five continents in five years. My most recent postcard came from Africa:

Feeling good, they have some amazing animals
here, miss you all!
Love, Emily

JULIE WALKER

I was in a bad fix. On the weekend I had transferred in a twenty-year-old female with aortic valve endocarditis. The referring cardiologist was from a small hospital in Connecticut. He said, "She had a bad cold, or upper respiratory infection. She went to bed and never woke up . . . her grandmother found her and couldn't arouse her and called 911. She came in completely comatose with a high fever . . . blood cultures grew out *staph aureus*, and we started triple antibiotic therapy. The fever came down, but she didn't wake up. The cardiac echo showed ugly vegetations on the aortic valve, and the brain CT showed a massive right-sided stroke. Her blood pressure was fine when she came in, but now the diastolic pressure is 30. Repeat echo shows 4+ insufficiency. She has been here three days, and there is nothing more we can do for her . . . we don't have a cardiac surgery program . . . will you take her in transfer?"

Instinctively, without thinking, I said, "Yes, send her . . . I have an open ICU bed." I hung up the phone, and almost immediately I had second thoughts about my willingness to take the transfer. The picture was not a good one. It sounded to me like this girl would need high-risk open-heart surgery to stay alive. The endocarditis had damaged her aortic valve, and the valve was leaking badly. She had at most twenty-four to forty-eight hours before the heart failure would lead to pulmonary edema. The fluid in her lungs would interfere with her oxygenation, and then she would die. The very high-risk open-heart operation was her only chance of survival.

I admitted her to our SICU and immediately repeated her cardiac echo. Indeed, she had 4+ aortic insufficiency, and the chest X-ray showed early pulmonary edema. If we were going to operate on her, we had to do it now. I called the Chief of Cardiac Surgery to discuss our options. He said, "If you don't operate, she will be dead by morning. If you do operate and she makes it through surgery, her head problem may be worse, not better. The heparin may increase the bleeding in her ischemic brain, and she may never wake up. What do you want to do? You are just starting your surgical career . . . and an early aortic valve death for you will not look good on the State Report in Albany, but it is up to you. No one will fault you for letting nature take its course. Her chances of having a meaningful recovery with the large size of her stroke are less than 10% . . . but it is your call."

He was trying to protect me and our surgical program. A surgical death in a twenty-year-old girl could prompt a Department of Health investigation. In this situation I was confident we would survive the review process, but a "state investigation" was never a good thing. It would look particularly bad for me as the operating surgeon.

I was agonizing about options when Jo, the SICU head nurse, found me in the back doctor's office. "The grandmother just arrived. She wants to talk to someone . . . do you want to talk to her, or do you want me to do it?" No one wants to deliver bad news— not the nurses or the ICU doctors—so I felt it was my job. She was in our hospital because I had transferred her in. She was my responsibility.

"Jo, can you bring her back here into the office? I will talk to her . . . "

I introduced myself to a large, serious-looking woman whose handshake told me she meant business. "I need someone to tell me what in the hell is going on with my granddaughter. I am her only family in the States . . . her mother lives in Canada. The doctors in the other hospital didn't do anything for her . . . they wouldn't even let her wake up. What are you going to do for her?"

I tried to explain that her granddaughter had an infection on a valve inside her heart. The infection was being treated with antibiotics, but it had caused a large stroke, and that was why her granddaughter was not awake and not moving. I said that the infection had also damaged a critical heart valve, and now her granddaughter, Julie, was going into heart failure. The doctors at the other hospital sent her to our medical center to possibly operate on her to remove the infected valve and replace it with a prosthetic valve. This was her only chance at survival. If we did nothing, her granddaughter would not make it through the night.

The grandmother looked shell-shocked. She was silent for a few seconds, and then she said, "If you do the surgery, what is her chance of waking up and returning to a normal life?"

I said, "Not more than 10–20%."

She then asked, "If you don't do the surgery tonight, she will not make it to the morning?"

"That is our opinion and the opinion of all the doctors who have seen her."

"Well, we don't have a choice, do we? Do the operation."

Despite the grandmother's eagerness, I was still uncomfortable with this decision. The chance of a good recovery was very poor. I thought I could replace the valve without a problem. That was the easy part, but the overall odds were bad. The CT scan of her brain was frightening. Her whole right brain looked severely damaged.

Pushing me toward surgery was the fact of her age. She was only twenty, a college junior. Young people can sometimes make remarkable recoveries from a serious neurological injury. And her grandmother was adamant. She again said, "When can you get started?"

I called my cardiovascular fellow and said, "Pre-op her . . . the grandmother will sign consent. Call the pump team and the on-call anesthesia attending . . . tell them we want to make the incision at midnight."

The cardiac surgery went surprisingly well. Her heart muscle had not been damaged by the infection and remained strong. The infected valve was completely incompetent with large, heaped-up vegetations that still contained bacteria. A sub-valvular abscess cavity was debrided and re-cultured. We were able to sew in a new biological valve prosthesis with no difficulty. Julie was weaned off the bypass machine with good ventricular functioning. The transesophageal echo demonstrated good valve mobility with no leakage. By 3:30 a.m. we had returned Julie to the SICU hemodynamically stable, with a well-functioning new aortic valve.

Now it was wait and see. I slept the rest of the night at my desk in the ICU, waiting for a catastrophe that never happened. There was no major bleeding, no cardiac arrhythmia, and no serious blood gas problems. Julie sailed through the night and the next three days like a routine heart case. The one major exception was that she did not wake up. She remained in a coma, so on the third post-op day I trached her to protect her ability to breathe safely. I made an incision on the lower part of her neck, removed the endotracheal tube from surgery, and placed a tracheostomy tube into the distal trachea. The tracheostomy tube guaranteed airway safety and comfort. This was routine protocol for patients who did not wake up after surgery or patients in a permanent coma.

Now, the most difficult work was about to begin. The recovery process would be slow and arduous. Julie remained in the SICU for two months. Two weeks post-op, she slowly started to open her eyes and respond to verbal commands. We placed a feeding tube that provided complete nutrition and calorie support. At four weeks, she could sit up and squeeze her right hand. Over time, she became more and more responsive to noise and the support staff. Most of the ICU patients were elderly, so the nurses loved focusing their attention on a twenty-year-old who was improving almost daily.

At the two-month mark, Julie could stand for short periods of time and respond appropriately to the nurses' questions. We removed her tracheostomy tube, and a month later she could ask questions and communicate in a meaningful way. The neurology service and rehabilitation team were seeing her daily and were thrilled with her progress. Three months after the surgery, she was transferred to the in-house rehabilitation floor. She relearned how to walk and talk over the next two months. She made dramatic progress, and six months post-op, she was discharged to her grandmother's house. She would continue outpatient rehab for the next two years and make an impressive neurological recovery.

I saw her biannually for the next two years and then referred her to a cardiologist in Connecticut. He saw her frequently and sent me notes that she was doing well and had returned to school. Julie completed a Bachelor of Science degree at NYU. She followed that with a Master's Degree in Biology, and she sent me a note saying she was working as a lab researcher at a nearby hospital.

Early one year, twelve years after her operation, Julie's cardiologist called me saying, "The valve is starting to leak on echo . . . it had looked good on prior yearly echoes, so this is a change. She has some shortness of breath . . . could you look at her?"

Julie came to my office, and I barely recognized her. She had been a girl at the first hospitalization, and now she was a mature woman. She had a little left-hand weakness but was fully active with a normal neurological exam. I was happy to see her, but unhappy to remind her that the pig biological valve in her heart had a finite life span of between ten and fifteen years. "Twelve years is a good result for an active young woman like yourself. We will need to operate and replace the valve, and this time we will put in a metal valve that will last twice as long or longer. You will have to take a blood thinner, but that is only one pill per day."

I told her this would be an elective operation for her. Unlike the last time, it was not an emergency, and she could do it whenever she desired in the next three months.

"This will be a much less risky operation compared to the first surgery. I think you will do very well. Most patients go home one week after surgery, and you can return to work three weeks later. Your shortness of breath will go away completely," I explained.

I was optimistic about this operation, remembering how sick Julie was at the first surgery. If she could recover from a massive stroke followed by open-heart surgery as well as she did, then this operation should be a "chip shot" for her and for us. I expected her to do well.

We made plans for the surgery. I discussed the operation with her grandmother, who was very worried that we had to do the operation "all over again." I explained that this elective surgery was much safer than last time. "Julie has not had a fresh stroke as she had before the first surgery. I expect her to do much better this time. This surgery is much less dangerous."

I would soon regret my optimistic words. Opening the skin and subcutaneous tissue was straightforward, but when we tried to divide the sternal bone with a bone saw, red blood suddenly gushed three feet into the air. I quickly pushed the sternum closed to stem the bleeding, but I knew we were in deep trouble. This was arterial blood that had to be coming from the aorta. There was no way I could proceed in the chest safely. She would bleed to death in two minutes.

I made my first assistant hold the chest closed. "Your only job is to push the sternal edges closed to stop the bleeding."

To anesthesia I said, "Get more blood in the room . . . I will cannulate the femoral artery and vein, and we will go on Fem-Fem Bypass. Then cool the patient to protect the brain." To the scrub nurse I said, "Get another fellow in the room to help me in the groin . . . I want to be on bypass in five minutes. Draw up the heparin, but don't give it till I say."

This was a crisis situation, but I had been here before. We needed to put cannulas in the femoral artery and vein so we could go on bypass. Then, we could cool the whole body to 20°C to decrease oxygen consumption in all the organ systems, especially the brain and heart. That would give us the freedom to open the sternum, isolate the heart, and control the bleeding aorta. All lost blood would be returned to the pump via special suckers connected to a reservoir.

We would be taking an uncontrolled situation and creating a safe environment to repair the aorta and insert a new aortic valve.

Once inside the chest cavity, I realized I could not clamp or occlude the aorta safely. Scar tissue from the first operation was dense, so I would need to turn off the pump completely and attach a Dacron graft to her aorta at the base of the arch vessels. This is a dangerous maneuver in any operation because the brain and all the organ systems would not have blood flow for about twenty minutes. To stop the blood flow to Julie's brain that had previous injury was particularly concerning, yet we had no choice, and we pushed ahead.

Over the next two hours we sewed an aortic graft to replace Julie's native aorta damaged by the saw. She only required twenty minutes of circulatory arrest. I then cut out Julie's porcine artificial valve that we had placed twelve years previously. I replaced it with a metal valve that usually would last twenty or more years. She would require lifelong blood thinners, but it was our most durable heart valve. We had protected the heart muscle with cardioplegia that cooled and stopped the heart from beating. By adding slush, the heart was less than 10° C during the valve replacement.

Our next task was to rewarm Julie to the normal 37° C. This took over an hour longer than usual because of our extensive cooling mandated by the circulatory arrest protocol.

There were no more surprises or problems in Julie's operation. Her first operation had been straightforward and uncomplicated. This operation was as difficult as an operation can be.

Six hours after skin incision, we returned Julie to the same ICU bed she had occupied twelve years previously. Two members of our ICU nursing staff remembered Julie well from her initial (very long) ICU stay. "She looks better now than she did twelve years ago. She is still young . . . we will take good care of her."

Surprisingly, Julie rebounded rapidly from this operation. Two days post-op, the nurses were helping her walk down the hall. Usually, some neurological defects from an original stroke would be expected to return after a second operation, but Julie's neurological exam remained normal. On post-op day fourteen, she was discharged to her grandmother's home.

I saw Julie two weeks after her discharge for a routine post-operative visit. She had no complaints, and her wound was healing well. She was taking the blood thinner for the new metal valve without problems. She was "looking forward" to returning to work.

Twenty years passed before I heard from Julie again. I assumed that she had moved to Canada to be with her mother and siblings. Her Coumadin (blood thinner) dosage was being followed by her cardiologist, but I had stopped hearing from him. I hoped she was well.

One day, I received a message that a "Julie Walker" had called and asked for an appointment. I had not forgotten her name or her history, but she was a stranger to my new office staff.

Julie came in looking like a fifty-year-old version of the girl I remembered well. I asked her how she was feeling and if she was still seeing her Connecticut cardiologist. "He checks my pro-time levels once a month, and everything seems good. My grandmother died five years ago, and I am living alone . . . still working part-time and doing child-care . . . I'm doing well."

A week later, I called her cardiologist to learn more. Patients do not suddenly reappear twenty years after heart surgery unless there is an issue they are worried about. He said, "I was planning to call you. Julie's valve is getting tight. Scar tissue must be growing into the annulus because her valve area is .9cm^2. Last year, it was 1.3cm^2 . . . she denies any symptoms, but .9 is tight. She will need a third operation."

So, there it was. Julie would need another operation thirty years after her original crisis. She wasn't ready to talk about it yet, but I think she wanted to look at me and see if I was still alive and operating. This was a bitter pill for her to digest, and I felt sorry for her.

Two months had passed when she called for another appointment, and she told my Patient Coordinator she wanted to see "her friend." She came in, and we talked about her work, her trip to Canada, and her nieces and cousins.

Finally, I said, "Julie, I spoke to your cardiologist. I know he told you what the last echo showed. Your valve is wearing out, and it will need to be replaced sometime in the next year. He and I agree that we can wait for symptoms to appear. So, promise to call me when you start to get shortness of breath going upstairs or when you see swelling in your ankles. Julie, you have this whole hospital in your corner. You have lots of friends here, and when the time comes, I promise we will get you through another operation safely."

Julie smiled.

FATHERS AND SONS

It was the new Millennium, the year 2000, when John Burke called me at my New York office. He said, "Karl, I've got a patient for you. He is Paul Harris, the son of the famous movie director Robert Harris, and he is having chest pain and shortness of breath when he plays tennis."

Robert Harris had won several Academy Awards, and I loved his films, which often featured large, beautiful land-scapes similar to Montana, where I grew up.

"His cardiologist has told him he needs to see a heart surgeon. He has a history of heart problems. He knows about you and wants to come to New York. Will you see him?"

I replied, "Sure, John, I can see him, but if he is having chest pain, he should go someplace closer. There are good heart programs in Seattle or Denver or Salt Lake City. I can give you the name of an excellent cardiac surgeon much closer to his home."

"No, he wants to come to New York. He says he is an old friend of one of your cousins, and he will feel more comfortable there." I was surprised by the fact that he would know one of my cousins, but we were from the same part of the country.

"Okay, John, give him my number, and tell him my secretary will arrange everything."

John said, "One last thing. He wants to play tennis with you at the tennis club. He has heard about the club from me, and I told him about your tennis."

I replied, "John, that may be inadvisable right now. Let me look at him first."

A week later, Paul Harris was sitting in my office talking nonstop.

"The truth is my father was not a big outdoorsman. Everyone thinks he was a great Western cowboy, but he wasn't. What he liked to do was make movies about the West. He did not like being in the elements. I have been an outdoorsman my whole life, much more than my father ever was, and I published three books about the technical aspects of elk hunting. I'll have my publisher send you some copies."

"Thanks. Now Paul, tell me about your heart."

"Well, I had a small heart attack three years ago, but I have been very active since then. I play tennis twice a week with friends like John. Every once in a while, I get a twinge of chest pain. I stop playing, and it goes away. My cardiologist says my EKG is okay, but I should check it with a stress test. What do you think?"

I replied, "I have already scheduled a stress test for tomorrow with one of our best cardiologists, Dr. Burke. He will go over your medical history, do a physical exam, and do the stress test in his office. If it is positive, we will order a cath the next day to look at your coronary arteries. Then he and I will review the films and come up with a game plan."

Paul interrupted, "If the stress test looks good, can we hit some balls at the tennis club? I brought my racquet."

I replied, "Absolutely, I will make a court reservation." The next day the stress test was strongly positive, and I told Paul, "Tennis is not an option. Tomorrow you are scheduled for a cardiac cath at 2:00 p.m. The cardiologist will inject dye into the coronary arteries and make a videotape of the blood flow. This will guide us on what next step to take. We might recommend medical therapy, or we might want to implant a stent in an area of blockage. If the disease is severe, we will recommend bypass surgery. The cath will also help us evaluate the strength of your heart muscle. That is a key finding. So, go to your hotel, talk to your wife, and return to the cardiac center at noon tomorrow. Dr. Burke and I will talk to you afterward."

The next day, Paul tolerated the cath procedure without a problem, but Dr. Burke and I were shocked when we reviewed the films. There are three coronary arteries that feed the heart muscle, and Paul had severe blockages in all of them. The disease was too widespread to treat with either stents or medical therapy. Surgery was the only good option. I told Dr. Burke, "I can put a graft to the LAD and the RCA, but that is all. The circumflex artery on the back is completely gone. That must be his infarct site from three years ago. Even the RCA is heavily diseased, and it is not a great target. What do you think?"

Dr. Burke was also disappointed and said, "The LAD is the only good target, but he does not have any better options . . . you have to operate."

Dr. Burke and I left the film viewing room and went to Paul's bedside. His wife, Anne, was holding his hand. I introduced Dr. Burke and myself and said, "I am happy that you are both here. We reviewed the films with the cathing cardiologist, and we are all in agreement that surgery is the best option . . . the blockages are too severe for an angioplasty procedure, and medications alone will not be adequate. We think surgery is the best path forward. I can do two bypasses. One will help a lot, and one target is not so good. The third artery is completely gone. That is the area of your infarct three years ago. What worries Dr. Burke and myself the most is that your ejection fraction is low. It measures the strength of your heart muscle. Normal is 50–60%, and yours is 20%. We hope the bypasses will increase the number to the 30–40% range. You can play tennis all day if it is 30–40%. Normally, bypass surgery carries a 1–2% risk, but in your case the risk is at least 10%. Your risk is higher because of your past infarct and the resulting weakness in the heart muscle. The worst complication of bypass surgery is a stroke, and that risk is 1%. This is a lot to absorb at once, so take your time thinking about what we have said, and Dr. Burke and I will return in a few minutes to answer your questions."

I wanted Paul and his wife to have some private time to discuss the information we had given them. Compared to most bypass operations, this was a high-risk case, and the upside of surgery was not great. He had only one good target, and his heart muscle was weak. If all went well, the operation would keep him alive for several more years. Not operating would be a death sentence; he would not survive another six months.

When we left the cath recovery room, I said to my colleague, "Do you have any other ideas of what we should do? That low ejection fraction of 20% doesn't give us much wiggle room if something goes wrong. What do you think?"

Dr. Burke, who was one of the senior staff cardiologists in the hospital, said, "He is 76, but he is a very active guy. If he wants to stay active, he must do the surgery. If he is content spending the rest of his life in an easy chair, reading and writing books, then we could hold off . . . let him decide."

When we returned to the post-cath holding area, I could see that Anne and Paul had made up their minds. Anne said, "We want to go ahead with the surgery . . . Paul is a very energetic guy, and he wants to stay that way. When can you do the operation?"

I said, "I know you have friends in the city. You can go for dinner over the weekend, but take it easy. We will admit Paul on Monday for surgery on Tuesday. My secretary will give you specific directions. If you have chest pain over the weekend, call my office, or come straight to the hospital emergency room, and they will contact me."

On Tuesday morning the anesthesia team put Paul to sleep without any difficulty or surprises. The transesophageal echo probe, placed in his esophagus, confirmed a poorly contracting ventricle consistent with the catheterization finding.

After prepping and draping, we made an eight-inch skin incision down the middle of his sternum. We opened the chest cavity and dissected the internal mammary artery off the chest wall. This conduit would be used to complete the bypasses to the LAD coronary artery, his best target. We took vein from his leg for the second bypass. After cannulation the heart-lung machine spun into action, and we were able to quickly arrest the heart with cardioplegia injected into the aortic root. I bathed the heart in iced slush, and when the myocardial temperature dropped to 10°C, we were ready to begin. I lifted the heart up and could see a large area of scar tissue on the back of the heart from the old infarction. I opened the small distal RCA, our first target. The lumen size was 1 mm, the lower limit acceptable for a bypass. I attached the vein graft using 8-0 Prolene, our finest suture material. I told my assistant that I expected the blood flow would be poor. "There is only a 50% chance this graft will be open a year from now."

The second bypass was made to the LAD vessel on the front of the heart. This was a good target, and the anastomosis to the IMA was completed without difficulty. The proximal end of the vein graft was sewn quickly to the ascending aorta. We vented air from the inside of the heart and removed the cross clamp.

To the perfusionist I yelled, "Warm."

The systemic blood had been cooled to 25° C, and it would take the pump 40 minutes to rewarm it to 37° C. The heart started contracting almost immediately despite being cold, which was a good sign.

When the rectal temperature reached 36° C, we gradually weaned off the bypass machine. Paul's heart was pumping vigorously, much better than before surgery. We measured the flow in the bypass grafts, and both were excellent. The ejection fraction that I had agonized about pre-op had increased from 20%–40%, a dramatic jump. "Let's close him and get him up to the intensive care unit." Three hours after the skin incision, Paul was transferred to the SICU, and I was ecstatic.

I told Anne, "He did as well as possible, actually much better than expected. I will not be happy until I see him wake up, but I am not expecting a problem neurologically. Our primary concern tonight is the risk of bleeding. There is a 5% chance he will have to go back to the OR, but usually I can predict bleeding, and I am not expecting a problem with him. He is very stable. After you see him, go back to the hotel. I will call you if there are any problems during the night."

I was very happy with our operation, and I predicted to our staff that Paul would do well. Another part of me, though, was worried and uncomfortable. Over the years,

I had heard about the Harris family reputation. It was no secret that the family was infamous for scandal. I had never thought much about it, but now it was making me uneasy.

Wednesday morning, the next day, Paul was awake and moving all his extremities. There were no neurological problems, and we extubated him. He said, "I feel great . . . when can we play tennis?" His heart function with the increased blood supply had improved significantly. When Anne came to visit, Paul was sitting on the edge of his bed and looked almost normal. He ate dinner on Wednesday night and looked well enough on Thursday morning that we transferred him to the step-down unit. There, he could sit up in a chair, watch television, and entertain guests. He could walk short distances with a telemetry monitor tracking each heartbeat. His progress was significantly better than I had anticipated for a seventy-six-year-old, and I was thrilled with his overall heart function.

On Friday, the nurses were walking Paul in the hallway. He was already asking about discharge plans, and I told him Monday would be the earliest possible date. He would have to stay in the New York area for two weeks so that I could observe his chest incision. "When you go back to Wyoming, no tennis, no shooting, and no exercise except walking for another month." He seemed okay with these restrictions. He said he was feeling "fine." I told him that Saturday was the first day of deer season in New York State, and I would be two hours away upstate, hunting. He smiled and said, "Shoot one for me." He casually mentioned that his youngest son,

Daniel, was flying into New York and would be visiting on Saturday. "I have not seen him in years . . . he lives in New Mexico, and I am very excited."

At 4:00 a.m. Saturday morning, I was speeding up the Taconic Parkway, heading north to my hunting territory near Hudson. I was always amazed at how fast one can escape from the city between 2:00 a.m. and 6:00 a.m. There was no traffic, and I knew I would arrive at my hunting cabin just before sunrise. I would have fifteen minutes to hike in the dark to my hunting blind. I wanted to be there before the first streaks of light pierced the eastern sky. In reality, I did not care much if I shot anything, but I liked being in the fall woods, and I liked looking for wild game. On the property I could see grouse, turkey, deer, and the occasional bear. And if I got lucky, I knew venison was heart-healthy compared to beef. The cabin was my getaway from the craziness and intensity of New York City.

At 10:00 a.m. I was on my way back to the cabin when my beeper went off. I hurried to the cabin where I had a landline and called the service. The operator said, "There is an emergency in the SICU. Dr. McGuinness called. I will patch you through to him."

While the operator was making the connection, I thought, *This is not good.* Dr. Cameron McGuinness was a second-year cardiovascular fellow, and if he had an ICU problem, he was supposed to call Dr. Godwin, the surgical attending on call for the weekend. I did not have any patients in the SICU.

Cameron McGuinness suddenly came on the line and said, "Karl, there is a big problem with Harris. He had a cardiac arrest on the floor. He looked fine on morning rounds. He had breakfast, and then his son came to visit, and the nurse said he suddenly became very emotional and confused. She checked his blood pressure and it had gone up to 240/100mmHg, and when he suddenly collapsed and passed out, they called a code. Dr. Godwin was in-house, and he and I arrived at the bedside about the same time. Harris had arrested and he had no blood pressure, so we opened his chest. The mediastinum was filled with blood, and there was bleeding from the aorta. We called a pump team STAT and rushed him with open-heart massage to the OR. We put him on bypass. He had ruptured an aortic suture line, probably from the hypertension. Dr. Godwin got the bleeding stopped, but the overall situation does not look good. The heart muscle is weak and is contracting poorly. Both of your grafts are open and have good flow, but the heart looks bad . . . I don't think he will make it. Dr. Godwin told me to scrub out and get a hold of you . . . it looks real bad."

I said, "Go scrub back in. Do everything you can to save him . . . I am three hours away . . . tell Liam to use his judgment. I am on my way."

I threw my gear into the back of the SUV, locked the cabin, and started the long haul back into the city. It sounded like Drs. McGuinness and Godwin had done everything possible to save Paul, but the prognosis was grim. The sudden increase in his blood pressure must have caused suture line bleeding. The blood and clot had compressed the heart, causing tamponade and cardiac arrest. The already weakened heart would have a difficult time tolerating this new insult.

When I got back to the hospital, Paul was in the SICU in critical condition. Anne had already been in to see him and was aware of his dire prognosis. I told her I did not think he would survive this final insult, and only four days later, despite all our efforts to save him, he passed away. He did not ever regain consciousness.

Anne held a small memorial service for Paul in the city two weeks later. It was well attended by his New York friends. At the close of the event, she handed me a handwritten note:

"There is a pocket knife from his father's most acclaimed film in the box—he brought it around everywhere. Thank you for trying to save my husband. We know you and your team did your best."

HIS ROYAL HIGHNESS

My routine on Wednesdays was to operate in the morning and see office patients in the afternoon. The patients were a mixture of pre-ops and post-ops. The post-ops were two to three weeks post-discharge and needed wound checks and medication reviews. For most, this would be their last visit with the surgical team, with further follow-up by the cardiologists. The pre-ops were being seen for the first time and were being evaluated for potential surgery. A cardiologist had decided the patient needed surgery, but the surgeon had to agree with the diagnosis and treatment plan. The post-operative patients were happy, optimistic, and relieved that their crisis was over. They were looking at a bright horizon. The pre-ops were anxious, full of questions, and pessimistic about their future. No one looked forward to heart surgery.

It was 1:00 p.m. on Wednesday afternoon. I had just completed a mitral valve operation and was taking off my gloves when Dr. Sam Jones came into the operating room. He was a cardiac anesthesiologist that I had known since medical school. He was a trusted friend, and we enjoyed working together. He said, "I know you are on your way upstairs to the clinic, but can I bother you for a minute?"

"We are having a problem in Room 16 . . . the surgeons have a retroperitoneal bleeding site that they cannot control. They keep packing the wound with laps to stop the bleeding, but they cannot keep it stopped. My team is having trouble keeping up with the blood loss at the head of the table. We have two big volume IV lines, and we have transferred eight units of blood, but the bleeding is not slowing down. The blood bank says they are running out of blood."

"Whose case is it? What did they do?"

"It's Wallace's case . . . and the patient is a serious big wig . . . he is actually some European prince."

"What? What is he doing here?"

"Well, it is supposed to be hush hush, but the prince has recurrent cancer. His first operation was three years ago in Europe. At first, he did well, but the cancer recurred . . . Wallace brought him to New York thinking we could do a better, more extensive operation here. He has five surgeons with him from Europe. The tumor is retroperitoneal down by the iliac vessels. I think they have punctured the iliac artery because the blood is very red . . . every time they take down the packing, they get flooded out. It has been going on for the last three hours without getting better, and the blood bank is scrambling to get more blood. Wallace told me to 'get help,' He said, 'Who is the best surgeon in the hospital at stopping bleeding?' Sorry, but I thought of you first . . . could you help us?"

Yikes, this was not good! Wallace was one of the best general surgeons in New York City. How was I going to fix something he couldn't fix?

I had heard several weeks ago that a VIP was being admitted, but I never guessed that it was a prince from Europe. What was I going to do in the OR that Dr. Wallace had not already done? His team could stop bleeding as well—or better—than myself, especially in the belly. In fact, the truth was that I had not operated in the belly in years. I didn't like the belly. I liked the chest . . . I was strictly a heart guy . . . not a belly guy.

"Could you just come and take a look? I told Wallace you are the best at stopping bleeding . . . " I suddenly felt skewered. What could I do?

"Okay, okay . . . I will take a look."

I followed Sam down the corridor to the General Surgery section of the operating rooms. I put on a new mask and gown and followed him into the OR.

There was a group of at least ten surgeons, medical doctors, or security people at the head of the table. Everyone was in scrubs, but I didn't see any faces I recognized. They stared at me like I was some kind of strange animal. Keith Wallace was on the surgeon's side of the operating room table with two assistants across from him. The patient looked massive under the drapes. I said, "How much does he weigh?"

Keith answered, "He is 250 pounds on a good day, when he is fasting. Thanks for coming in. We have bleeding down in the pelvis . . . with all the fat, the exposure is terrible. I think I got all of the recurrent tumor out . . . there is a mass of lymph nodes, and everything is bleeding . . . it's arterial and venous. We are running out of blood . . . can you give us a hand?"

What could I say? The last thing I wanted to do was get involved in a case like this, but Keith Wallace was a good guy and an excellent surgeon. If our roles were reversed, I thought he would scrub in and help me. With the audience at the head of the table, he had to be feeling a huge amount of pressure. And the last thing our hospital needed was for the world to know that a prince bled to death in our OR. That we could not tolerate. Even if it took all the king's horses and all the king's men to put the prince back together again—we had to stop the bleeding. And as Wallace was speaking, an idea was coming together in the back of my mind as to how we might be able to get the job done.

"Okay . . . okay . . . Sam, can you get a cell saver from the Cardiac OR and set it up in here? Keith, we are going to recycle the lost blood back into the patient as we do routinely in Cardiac . . . I will get one of my fellows to work with me, and we will have our own perfusionist for the recycle machine. We run the risk of recycling tumor cells, but that is better than bleeding to death. Are you okay with that?"

He answered, "Okay."

"I will run to the dressing room and change my scrubs . . . Sam, are you okay with the plan?"

Sam nodded.

In the locker room I called my office and told my staff to reschedule as many appointments as possible. "I doubt I will be available until after 5:00 p.m. If some patient wants to wait, that's okay, but I could be stuck down here for four or five hours."

Dr. John Addison, the cardiovascular fellow on my service, ran into the locker room. "Our patient from today is doing well in the CICU (cardiac ICU). The vital signs are stable, there is minimal bleeding, and the cardiac output is five liters. What's going on here?"

"I have a gift for you. For as long as it takes, you have to help me try to save a prince! It could take three hours or ten hours; but you and I are not going to let this royal old man die in our OR . . . are you okay with that?"

I told John the whole story, "This is not going to be easy . . . we have to get the bleeding under control. We will have a cell saver to recycle the lost blood as in a heart case, but we have to find a way to stop the blood loss. It may be arterial blood from an iliac artery injury. I hope you are feeling strong. The patient is 250 pounds, and the exposure will be terrible."

The cell saver was new technology only used by the cardiac surgery service. We could suck up lost blood, filter out nonhematologic particles like fat, and re-transfuse it in minutes. We used it routinely in every cardiac surgery case, but it had not been used in general surgery. It would allow us to be very aggressive about looking for the bleeding sites and then stopping the blood loss. All lost blood would be recycled back into the patient via Sam's transfusion lines.

When we scrubbed in, there was not only the gallery watching at the head of the table, but word had gotten around the OR, and multiple other surgeons were crowding into our room and looking over our shoulders. Normally, I do not get nervous in the OR, but this was not my OR . . . this was not my normal venue. For the first time in my life, I felt quite uncomfortable, and I started to perspire. I said to the scrub nurse, "Manuel, I will need felt pledgets of all different sizes loaded on 2-0 Prolene needles. I am going to be sewing fast, so you may need another scrub nurse to help you. I am going to place felt all over the pelvis and the retroperitoneum. It is going to be a bloody mess, but we are going to stop the bleeding. John, you are going to be sucking blood all the time. I don't want to lose any red cells. You also have to tie knots for me and give me exposure. It will not be easy. The two things we cannot do is to occlude the iliac arteries completely and we cannot occlude or injure the ureters . . . okay?"

John and I dove into the retroperitoneum, and three hours later we were done. We had all the pelvic bleeding stopped. The patient's retroperitoneum looked like a felt garden with pledget material planted all over the posterior abdominal cavity. The patient's blood pressure had been stable throughout because Sam and his team had recycled all the lost blood back into the prince's intravenous lines. The prince had pulses in both feet, so I knew I had not damaged his iliac arteries, and there was a liter of urine in his Foley bag. The kidneys and the ureters had also avoided injury and were doing their job. Sam announced that he had recycled eleven units of cell saver blood, approximately twice the prince's total blood volume. "Thank you, Sam . . . he will probably need fresh frozen plasma and platelets to help with hemostasis."

To Keith I said, "I think you can probably close. If he bleeds tonight, John and I will take him back and start all over again. I think I would place Jackson-Pratt drains down into the pelvis for twenty-four hours but not much longer. There is a lot of felt in the retroperitoneum. If he gets infected, he is probably a dead man."

With that warning, Keith shook John's and my hand. "Thank you for the help . . . that cell saver was a life-saver for the prince. We still need to create a colostomy and close his belly. I cannot thank you enough."

John and I were exhausted but thrilled to have been able to help. Out of the operating room I said, "John, check our post-op from today . . . be sure he is not bleeding . . . and then come to my office. You can help me see the clinic patients that have stuck around. Then we can both go home. We have had enough fun for one day."

The prince survived his operation without further problems. As we anticipated, he had a prolonged post-operative course in the ICU, but one month later he returned to Europe feeling significantly better. He resumed his responsibilities in his country and continued his close relationship with the United States president.

Two years later, not surprisingly, he developed a second recurrence of his tumor with metastatic disease to his pancreatitis and kidneys. He elected to return to the United States for supportive care supervised by Dr. Wallace, and he eventually passed away surrounded by his family (which included his five children) at our hospital at the age of eighty-five.

A CORNER ROOM

I knew there was a problem with Henry. He normally played squash three times a week at our tennis club, but I had not seen him on the courts for several months. Instead, I was told he was swimming laps in the club pool. In the twenty years that I had known him, I had never seen Henry in the pool. He was not a swimmer; he was a squash player.

I asked Peter, the head tennis pro, "What's up with Henry?"

Peter said, "He told me he was taking up swimming to stay in shape . . . he said he is backing off on squash . . . I am not sure what is really going on with him."

I asked, "Is his hip bothering him? He hurt it six months ago."

"No, I don't think so . . . he didn't give me an explanation."

Something was not right with Henry, and an alarm went off in my head. Henry was a childhood diabetic who developed severe coronary artery disease (CAD). Ten years previously, I had done a quadruple coronary artery bypass operation on Henry's heart. He recovered rapidly and resumed playing competitive squash two months later.

It is well known that a diabetic who has had bypass surgery can develop recurrent blockage in their bypass grafts five to ten years after their operation. This occurs even if they strictly control their diet and take their medications. Maybe Henry was experiencing chest pain when he played squash but not when he was swimming. I had seen this scenario before.

I called Jim Howe, Henry's cardiologist at the hospital, and told him my concern about Henry. He said, "I don't think he is having a problem with his heart. He had a normal stress test three months ago. On echo his left ventricle is still strong . . . what he complains about the most to me is his renal failure. As you know, he started dialysis three years after bypass surgery, and he has never gotten used to his dialysis routine. Actually, I think he hates the dialysis. He has never become comfortable lying in a bed in the middle of the day for three to four hours at a time. And he has dialysis three times a week. In addition, he hates being stuck with needles."

Dr. Howe paused and then continued, "Until recently, he has been very active with both his squash and his business schedule, but lately, the dialysis seems to cramp his style both mentally and physically. I think he feels 'crippled' for the first time in his life, and I think he is depressed. I may start him on an antidepressant."

I immediately felt bad for Henry. It had been a long, slow fall from grace. Born in Florida, he had been a child prodigy in squash. He was a U.S. junior squash champion from the age of fourteen. He was also one of the first diabetic athletes to successfully compete at an international level, which included deep runs at the British Open Squash Championships, otherwise known as the "Wimbledon of Squash." He was a trailblazer for all diabetics in professional sports. He was also an excellent student with an "A" grade average in his four years at Stanford. For the last twenty-five years, he'd been a successful ad executive in NYC, and he continued playing competitive club squash in the NYC area.

When I joined my tennis club, I was one of the lucky new members who Henry took under his wing. He decided he could improve my game, as he was also an excellent tennis player. He soon became my unofficial coach. For the next ten years, he encouraged me, challenged me, and coached me to become a better player. Together, we won many club tournaments, and I was not alone—there were many other players that he encouraged and coached. I think that at a very profound level he loved racquet sports, and he wanted to share that love. For many years he was the brightest star at the club, and he shared his light with all of us.

Now that enthusiastic light was starting to fade. At age seventy-two, he stopped playing squash because the dialysis had exhausted him both mentally and physically. Maybe

Henry's cardiologist was right. Maybe he was clinically depressed. Living with diabetes for a lifetime had been a challenge, but the reality of living with chronic renal failure and dialysis had become too much.

It was time for me to have a talk with my friend. I called Henry and asked if we could meet for lunch at the club. When Henry entered the dining room of the club two days later, I hardly recognized him. He had lost at least twenty pounds and looked gaunt. Henry had always been robust and hearty but now looked depleted; he looked exhausted. We shook hands and I had to help him into a chair. We ordered lunch and I said, "Henry, what is going on with you? I have not seen you on the court for months. I heard you had stopped playing squash . . . how come?"

He answered, "I cannot play anymore . . . I cannot see the ball because of the glare of the indoor lighting, or maybe the diabetic retinopathy is finally getting to me. I cannot see well enough to make the ball hit the center of my racquet, and equally, or more problematic, I cannot run on the court. I have an infected toe, probably caused by diabetes, and I cannot cover the court. I also have generalized weakness. I have lost weight, and the dialysis and renal failure cause me to feel tired all the time. You know the dialysis is three times a week, three hours each session, and it has become an exhausting routine over the last couple of years. I hate it. I am frustrated, and I feel like I have had enough. My wife Veronica keeps insisting that I go to all my dialysis sessions, but I feel like I cannot take it anymore.

I said, "I know the dialysis is hard, no one likes dialysis, but with your kidneys it is mandatory. It has kept you alive over the last six years, and it has kept you on the squash court. You are still one of the best players in the club. Your toe will get better eventually, and we can buy you sunglasses to cut the glare from the indoor lights. You cannot stop now."

"Well, what would happen if I did stop the dialysis? What exactly would happen?"

"The urea and potassium would build up in your blood to dangerous levels. You would slowly get weaker and weaker, and when the potassium level rose high enough, your heart would stop beating."

"Is it painful?"

"Usually not."

"How long would it take?"

"I don't know exactly, but probably four to five days."

"And then, that is it . . . I would be dead?"

"Yes, and we don't want that."

"Well, I appreciate your sentiments, but I have been thinking a long time about this, and I have also been talking with Veronica. I feel bad and weak almost all the time. I have lost 80% of my strength. I have become exhausted just walking two blocks from my apartment to the club today. For the last month I have not felt well enough to go to my office. My kids are in Seattle. I have almost stopped eating. I ask myself what I am living for?"

Henry hesitated and took a deep breath. "To make matters worse, I think I must be a pain in the ass to live with. I feel sorry for Veronica. Thank God she still has a job and goes to her office each day . . . she can get away from me for part of the day."

I could tell that Henry wanted to vent, so I did not interrupt him.

"You know . . . what I have been thinking about . . . I almost called you last week."

I nodded.

"Could you admit me to the hospital? Put me in a corner room like I had after the bypass operation. A room where I could look out and see the city . . . you could stick an IV in my arm and keep me hydrated and then stop the dialysis. You said I would last three to four days. I would have a bottle of gin, some ice and tonic, and I would invite all my New York friends for a "last drink and last visit" . . . all very civilized. Veronica can come and go when she wants. She wouldn't have to worry about me . . . she trusts you and your staff. That would be a very civilized way to die, don't you think? Could you arrange that for me?"

When playing a doubles tennis match with Henry, he would always have a "plan" of how to win, and we would talk about it before the first serve. I wasn't surprised that he had a plan on how to choreograph his own death.

"Henry, you know I would do anything for you. We have been friends for a long time, but I want you and Veronica to think about this for a while longer. Wait at least five days before you make a final decision. Keep up the dialysis in the meantime. After five days if you both want to go ahead with the plan, I will get you a corner room. You better let your children know."

"Between now and then, I will talk to your nephrologist. To refuse dialysis is your decision, and I will let the hospital know of your decision. If you have questions or change your mind, let me know, and we can talk more about it."

On a Friday night, ten days later, I admitted Henry to the cardiac step-down unit. He had a large corner room with a refrigerator and a small serving table. For the next forty-eight hours, there was a constant stream of old friends from the club, business associates from the city, and other close friends. His children flew into town and spent the daylight hours with their father. On Sunday night Henry started to fade. He was arousable but slept most of the time. He was not in pain. Veronica and I stopped the parade of guests, and on the fourth night he passed away. The last garbled words he said to me were, "Be sure to stay relaxed on the tennis court." He was my tennis coach to the very end.

Veronica organized a memorial service at a city church, and three hundred people crowded into the service. There were several memorial speakers, and I was honored to make the last comments.

"Henry was an outstanding individual. It was a privilege to have known him and an honor to consider him my friend. He was an inspiration and a role model for me and many others in this room. The light that Henry leaves behind will guide my path and the path of many others for years to come."

SIGNOR RICCIO

I was working in my office late on a Saturday night when my beeper went off. I called the service, and the operator said, "Dr. Holmes wants you to call him STAT on Braum 3. He has an emergency."

I didn't like the sound of that, especially since I was not the on-call cardiac surgeon. I was writing a textbook, and I had a deadline in three months. Saturday nights were my best and often only guaranteed work time, usually without interruptions. Ben Holmes was a cardiac fellow, and if he had a patient care problem, he was supposed to notify the on-call attending, not me.

Braum 3 was the step-down unit for post-cardiac surgery patients who had graduated from the ICU and would soon be discharged home. They were our most healthy patients, not our "problem" patients.

I called Braum 3, and the clerk said, "Dr. Holmes is standing next to me. I will pass the phone."

"Ben, what's up?"

He said, "I know you are not on call . . . I know you are working on your book . . . but I have a big problem, and I need your advice."

"A seventy-five-year-old man who is ten years post-mitral valve replacement was admitted tonight to Braum 3. He is in severe congestive heart failure. He was told six months ago by his cardiologist that his prosthetic valve was both stenotic and incompetent. He was told it needed replacing. He is now in severe failure and is very short of breath. He was admitted through the emergency room, and he does not look good." Ben hesitated and caught his breath.

"His cardiologist is Ian Raymond . . . *the* Ian Raymond . . . and his daughters have been calling his office all day, but without success. The daughters did not know what to do, so they brought him to our emergency room. I know that Ian refers all his surgical cases to the Chief, but when I called Dr. Isaac's home, I get the answering machine. I called his service, but they could not find him. I don't know what to do . . . can you look at him with me? He looks sick, he looks like he could die anytime, and I think he is a VIP."

I said, "Ben, you did the right thing. Call the surgical ICU and tell them you need a bed . . . I am on my way down."

I ran for the Braum 3 elevator. It was old and slow, but I needed time to think. If this was one of Ian Raymond's patients, he was a VIP by definition. Dr. Raymond was the best-known cardiologist in our hospital, and probably the most recognized cardiologist in all of New York City. He had published several best-selling medical books for the lay public; he had his own weekly radio show, *Ask Dr. Raymond*; and he reportedly took care of several ex-presidents. He had the largest VIP cardiology practice in the city, and when patients required surgical care, he referred only to chiefs of service like our own boss, Dr. Isaac.

Ben met me at the elevator and walked me to the patient's bedside. "We can get an ICU bed, and the nurses are setting up now."

The patient looked chronically ill and was struggling with each breath. With one look, I knew he would need to be intubated. I introduced myself and said, "We are moving you to intensive care. We will give you some sedation and put a tube in your throat. It will make your breathing easier. We will try to keep you comfortable. Do you understand me?" He slowly nodded and closed his eyes.

I turned to the nurses, "What are his vital signs?" The bedside nurse handed me a clipboard and I read, "Heart rate 120, irregular, blood pressure 80/50mmHg, respiratory rate 35, O_2 Sat 55%." His pulse was very irregular.

I said, "Ben, call the ICU and tell them we are on our way. Tell the charge nurse to have an intubation tray set up. I will also pass a Swan-Ganz catheter and an arterial line. I want an intra-aortic balloon pump set up at the bedside. Tell the nurses this man is very sick and could arrest at any moment."

Two nurses brought a stretcher to the bedside, and the four of us lifted the patient carefully onto it. We took the back elevator down to the surgical ICU, where we could safely take care of him. I was confident we could temporarily stabilize the patient and, with sedation, keep him more comfortable. I was most worried about his breathing. He couldn't keep breathing at a rate of 35 for long. I injected 4mg of morphine into his IV line and carefully passed an endotracheal tube into his mouth and down into his trachea. I placed a needle into his left subclavian vein and threaded a Swan-Ganz catheter through his right side of his heart and into his pulmonary artery. The pulmonary pressure was 80/40, twice as high as expected. The malfunctioning prosthetic mitral valve was the culprit. It was both narrowed and leaking. It would need urgent replacement to keep him alive.

The patient tolerated these procedures without a fall in his blood pressure, so I felt safe giving him additional morphine to keep him comfortable. Next, I quickly placed an intra-aortic balloon pump, a heart support device, in the femoral artery. It would support the work of his failing heart and temporarily stabilize his condition until we decided on a definitive treatment plan.

I glanced at the clock on the ICU wall. It was midnight. Our patient was stable for now, but the balloon pump was only a temporary fix. His chance of surviving until the morning was less than 10%. It was time to find Dr. Isaac.

I dialed his home number in Connecticut, and he picked up on the first ring. I told him our saga, and I emphasized that this was Dr. Raymond's patient. He said, "I know this man. Ian told me about him several months ago. I haven't met him yet, but he owns a famous Italian clothing store in Manhattan, and it's the best in the city. It is famous. He has two daughters. Have you talked to them?" I said, "No, but Ben says one of them is in the waiting room. I wanted to talk to you first."

He said, "It sounds like he has to be done tonight. I am two to three hours away, and you can do the surgery as well as I can . . . tell the daughters that I am out of town and am not available. Be sure Ben locates the cath films. He is supposed to be without coronary disease, but look for yourself. Call me in the morning. And one more thing . . . leave a message for Raymond when you finish the case. Good luck!"

I had always appreciated Dr. Isaac's confidence in me. He was the Chief of Cardiac Surgery at the hospital, but he had never shied away from assigning me the hardest cases. I liked the challenge, and the way I looked at it, without the surgery the patient was dead. With the surgery, we had a shot at saving him. It was time to find his family.

Ben said, "Both daughters are now in the family waiting room."

I said, "Let's go talk to them . . . you come with me."

Two middle-aged women were the only family left in the waiting room. I introduced Dr. Holmes and myself, and I summarized the events of the evening. I said, "Dr. Holmes realized how sick your father was, he called me, and together we have temporarily stabilized him. He has a heart support device in place that is keeping him alive. I have spoken to Dr. Isaac on the telephone, and he agrees that without emergency surgery, your father will not survive the night. Dr. Isaac cannot come in, and he wants Dr. Holmes and me to operate as soon as possible. The surgery is high risk, in the 20–30% range. That gives him a 70% chance of coming through okay. The worst complication of heart surgery is a stroke, and that risk is 2–3%. Again, if we do nothing, he will not survive. He is not passing any urine, and without immediate surgery his kidneys will shut down completely. You will have to sign consent. Do you have any questions?"

Both daughters looked numb and said nothing. Finally, the older sister said, "He loves our store. What are the chances he will be able to come back to work? It is his whole life . . ."

I said, "Chances are good. I am guessing, but at least 60% for the good. If the surgery goes well, he could go back to work with the same energy he had five years ago."

The sisters looked at each other and the older one said, "How soon can you start . . . where do we sign consent?"

I had no trepidation about doing the surgery. It would be a long, hard slog of an operation because he was a re-op, he was old, and there would be scar tissue plastered all around his heart. I often told resident doctors that re-ops were twice as hard as primary cases and sometimes twice as long. Skin to skin, a first-time mitral valve replacement is completed in under three hours. This man was seventy-five, he was in severe congestive heart failure, and he was not passing urine.

He would take at least five to six hours. On the upside, we had a heart support device, the balloon pump, already in place, and that would help dramatically. The alternative, no surgery, carried a 100% mortality.

When we transferred Mr. Riccio to the ICU, Ben had called the OR and told the nurses to set up a cardiac room, and he asked that the on-call anesthesia team be called in. They were now ready, and they helped Ben and the ICU nurses transfer our patient to the OR. I ran down to the cath lab and reviewed Mr. Riccio's cath study done six months before. Despite what I assumed, Signor Riccio had beautifully clean coronary arteries. No bypasses were required.

The operation went as well as a difficult re-operation could go. It took us two hours to dissect the scar tissue off the heart so I could approach the mitral valve safely. We initiated cardiopulmonary bypass and arrested the heart without difficulty. I opened the left atrium, which was twice the normal size, and I had good exposure of the ten-year-old prosthetic valve. It was heavily calcified and obstructed, but I resected it without complications. I placed a new Carpentier-Edwards porcine prosthesis into the mitral orifice and closed the atrium. I de-aired the heart and reestablished coronary perfusion of the heart muscle.

We weaned Signor Riccio off the bypass machine easily. The heart support device placed in the ICU reduced the workload of the heart dramatically. We gave protamine to promote coagulation, but it still took Ben and me two hours with the electrocautery to stop the bleeding. While closing the sternal bone, the anesthesiologist happily announced "He is making urine . . . his kidneys are coming back."

At 6:00 a.m. we removed the drapes and transferred Mr. Riccio back to the surgical ICU. Our outstanding ICU nurses took over his care, and I exhaled completely. Ben and I felt we had won a victory.

As soon as Signor Riccio had stabilized, I asked Ben to run upstairs and bring his daughters to the ICU. The nurse told me they had spent the night in the waiting room; they had never gone home. When they came in, I took them to his bedside and said, "Overall, everything went well, no surprises. I will not be happy until I see him wake up and move his arms and legs, but I am not anticipating a neurological problem. His cardiac function has improved dramatically, and the new valve is working well. I do not expect him to wake up until this evening or tomorrow morning, so you should go home and get some sleep. Dr. Holmes or I will call you if any problems come up. The operation went better than we expected."

There was suddenly a commotion at the front desk of the ICU. Dr. Raymond burst into the unit saying, "Well, where is he?" The head nurse brought him to the bedside, where I could tell he recognized the daughters. He shook hands, and without looking at Signor Riccio or his chart, he said, "Everything went well with your father's surgery. When I got your message last night, I immediately called my surgeon, Dr. Krieger. He is our best surgeon for re-operations like this. Your father will be fine."

Signor Riccio tolerated his post-operative course exceedingly well. When he woke up the following day, we removed the breathing tube without any problems. Feeling much better, he quickly returned to being what his daughters called his "normal self." He was a delightful Italian man, energetic and grateful for his medical care. Two weeks after the surgery, he insisted on walking out of the hospital on his own, with an arm around each of his devoted daughters.

Three weeks later, he returned to my office for his post-op visit, and he looked full of energy. He insisted that my wife and I visit their beautiful store on Madison Avenue. When he showed us his store, he said, "This is *my* operating room."

We had a wonderful visit and were graciously given exquisite cashmere scarves.

"As long as I live, I want you and your wife to come yearly to enjoy a gift from Italy . . . I insist . . . it is part of the deal."

We visited the store one more time the following year, and again Senior Riccio was overly generous with beautiful gifts from his store. Out of embarrassment, we did not return, but we exchanged Christmas cards, and he kept me posted on his health.

Signor Riccio ran his store for fifteen more years and died in his nineties. The daughters have continued the business and have renamed it after their father.

THE "BIG DOG"

Nancy, my office manager, grabbed me as soon as I walked through the front door. "Bill Cobb called from another hospital . . . he has called twice. He is in the CCU with a patient for transfer. The patient arrested during a stress test yesterday. I will get him on the line."

I had just finished an aortic dissection repair and was looking forward to sitting down for a moment when Nancy handed me the phone. She nodded her head expectantly as if to say, "Don't get too comfortable in that chair, Mister."

"Hello Bruce, what can I do for you?" I had worked closely with Bruce for three years after he finished his cardiology fellowship. He was a good doctor, and I trusted his judgment. He had recently taken over the directorship of the CCU at another hospital, and I was happy for his promotion.

He answered, "I have a sixty-two-year-old real estate developer who was having a routine stress test in his private cardiologist's office when his heart fibrillated. The cardiologist said that in twenty years of doing stress tests, he had never used the defibrillator paddles, and he was slow to hook them up. The patient fell down and hit his head. Finally, the cardiologist shocked him, and the developer converted to sinus rhythm. The doctor quickly called 911 and had the patient shipped to the nearest hospital."

Dr. Cobb continued, "I was here when he came in . . . he was confused but with a good rhythm, and he gradually cleared mentally during the night. His EKG showed anterior ischemia. He is moving all extremities, and I think his head will be okay. We cathed him this morning, and he has triple vessel disease and a 90% left main. He has three good targets for you to bypass. He has a younger spouse who was here all night. She says you operated on several of their friends. She wants to move him to your hospital for the surgery. I know you have a full schedule, but could you squeeze him in tomorrow?"

I said, "Send him over, we will make an ICU bed and put him on the schedule. We will also get a neuro consult. Is there anything else that I need to know about him?"

Bruce hesitated for a minute and then he said, "Well, I have gotten at least five outside phone calls about this guy. I think he must be a very high-profile developer in the New York area . . . a big dog in the city."

"Thanks, Bruce . . . we like big dogs. I will make a bed now. Send him by ambulance, and thank you for the referral. I will keep you posted."

The big dog's name was Allan Rose, and although he did not at first glance look much like a "big dog," he would eventually live up to that description. He was small in stature, maybe 5' 7' and 157 pounds, and visibly exhausted from the cardiac episode.

His spouse, Maxine, did all the talking. "I've been telling him to see a doctor for months—he has been having chest pain every day—but he didn't listen to me. I knew he wasn't right, and now this. Can you help him, please?"

I said, "We can help him, but first we are ordering a CT scan of his head to make sure he did not bleed into his brain. If it is all right, we will operate tomorrow afternoon. He needs three or four bypasses. The operation will take four hours, and I will talk to you when it is over. The operative risk is 3–5%, with a 2% risk of neurological injury. Will you speak to the rest of his family?" She looked me straight in the eye and said, "I will speak to all of them."

The operation the next day went well. I was able to complete four bypasses with excellent target vessels. I can usually predict who will do well post-op based on the quality of the target vessels and the quality of the conduit (veins and arteries) that I use for the bypasses. This patient had excellent conduit and excellent targets. His heart muscle had not been damaged by the arrest in his cardiologist's office, so his overall prognosis was excellent. He boomed off the bypass machine like a patient half his age. I knew he would do well.

I found Maxine waiting alone in the family room, and I gave her the good news. "He is going to be fine . . . he has the heart of a thirty-year-old. After you see him tonight, go home and get some sleep. You cannot do anything for him here. Don't come back until 1:00 p.m. tomorrow. If all goes well, he will be awake by then. If there are any problems during the night, I will call you. After 8:00 a.m. tomorrow morning, you can call Nancy in my office for an update. Stay strong . . . he is going to do well." I gave her a brief hug and went back to the ICU.

Some lucky people breeze through open-heart surgery, and Allan was one of those people. At 10:00 a.m. the next morning, he was awake, and the ICU staff extubated him. When Max returned at 1:00 p.m., Allan was talking as if he had a hernia repair. He said, "Max, they gave me some morphine, and I have no pain at all." The following day, we transferred him to the step-down unit and removed his central lines. He was able to stand up unassisted, and on post-op day three, he was walking in the hallway with Maxine. On post-op day five, I allowed Max to take him home, with strict instructions about no weightlifting and daily ambulation. With Max's help and support, he had a perfect post-op course, and he returned to his office work four weeks after the surgery.

During the next two months, I checked on Allan and Max several times. Their residence in the city was on my way home from the hospital and only three blocks from my apartment. They lived in a duplex at the top of an apartment building overlooking the East River. He had a private elevator that whisked me upstairs, and we would sit and eat and drink on the outdoor terrace while watching the boats on the East River. Over the next twelve months after his surgery, we became friends. We both played tennis, we both skied in Aspen where he had a second home, and his country house in Southampton was four blocks from my modest summer residence. A mutual friend described Allan and Max's Southampton estate as "more of a small college campus than a private home." Over the next two decades, we played tennis in the summer, and we skied in the winter. We became very close friends.

Not long after the heart surgery, Allan and Max had a beautiful baby girl, and our children became playmates.

Over the next twenty years, Allan's construction business flourished. He built hotels, apartment complexes, and large office buildings on the East Coast between Boston and New Orleans. He worked hard and was constantly traveling. During the few times we had dinner together alone, he would reflect on his past life. "For a boy from Brooklyn, who never went to college, I did all right. My first job in construction after high school was driving a dump truck. I drove for three years before I moved up a bit in the company and started helping my boss bid on construction jobs."

I made sure Allan kept up his yearly cardiology appointment. He was seeing an excellent cardiologist, Dr. Pappas, who did yearly stress tests and sent the reports to me. They had looked excellent, so I was surprised when Allan, after returning from an Aspen skiing trip, made an urgent call to my office. He wanted to meet for dinner. He said it was for "just the two of us" at Wolf's, two blocks from his apartment. We met, and I could immediately detect an unusual urgency or fear in his behavior. He said, "I just flew back from Aspen in our company plane, and I almost didn't make it. I got so short of breath I thought I would die. I had to lie down on the floor of the plane. The stewardess gave me oxygen to breathe, or I wouldn't have made it home. I saw Dr. Pappas today and he did a stress test that was normal, and he did an echo. He said that my aortic valve is narrowed, but it doesn't need surgery yet. What do you think?"

I responded, "Allan, it is not normal for you to be short of breath . . . come to my office tomorrow at 1:00 p.m., and we will repeat the echo. Maybe the valve is worse than Dr. Pappas thinks."

The echo the next day showed a valve area of 1.1cm^2. I told Allen, "We normally don't operate unless the valve is less than 1.0cm^2, but you are eighty, and if you want to stay active with skiing and tennis, I think it should be replaced. The good news is that we can now replace your valve without opening your chest. There is new technology . . . I will give you reading information about it. It is a great procedure—no incision, no pain. Two days in the hospital and you can go back to work. It is called TAVR – Trans Aortic Valve Replacement. It is perfect for you."

Allan and I had dinner on Monday, and we placed the new TAVR valve on Thursday. The day prior to the procedure, we did a cardiac cath that showed his twenty-year-old bypass grafts were all open and functioning well. Allan went home on Saturday, and like most workaholics, he returned to his office on Monday.

Three weeks later, Allan called my office to set up another dinner. Again, he asked if "just the two of us" could meet at Wolf's. He arrived early, and when I walked in, he bounded out of his chair to shake my hand. "I feel the best I have felt in the last five years. I played tennis yesterday, and it was the best tennis I have played in the last ten years . . . that new valve makes me feel like a new man. I feel like I am young again."

He paused for a moment, and then he said, "I want to make a donation to your department at the hospital. What do you think?" I smiled and said, "That is fantastic, Allan, extremely generous of you . . . our department and the hospital will be thrilled. You know you don't have to do this, but thank you very much."

Allan did well for the next five years, and I saw him a couple of times a year socially. I assumed all was stable until late in August on a very hot Saturday afternoon, Maxine called our summer house. She said, "Karl, can you come over here? Allan does not look good. He has been taking a tennis lesson. You know Pavlo, the Polish tennis pro he likes? They have been hitting for an hour, and Allan fell down. He looks bad. He's slurring his speech."

I raced the four blocks to their home. This did not sound good. It was 90°F in the shade—not a good day for a tennis lesson.

Allan was lying down next to the tennis court with a drink of water in his hand. He looked at me with a slight smile as if he knew he had made a mistake. I felt his radial pulse, which was weak and thready and over 100 beats per minute. I said, "Lie down flat," and I felt his groin pulse. The systolic pressure was 80 to 90. I made Allan move both his arm and legs to command. I took the pro aside and said, "Are you trying to kill him? He is 85! Dead clients don't look good on your resume . . . and they stop taking lessons." I went back to Allan and said, "Drink as much Gatorade as you can, stay in the shade, and we will move you inside the house."

I walked with Max into the house and told her, "He is dehydrated, and his blood pressure is low. We have two choices. We can call 911 and take him by ambulance to Southampton Hospital. There, we can give him IV hydration in the emergency room. Or we can carry him into the air-conditioned bedroom, and you can resuscitate him with Gatorade. I think we can go the Gatorade route, but if he passes out you call 911, okay?" She nodded.

The pro and I lifted Allan onto a chair and carried him into the air-conditioned bedroom. We put him on top of the bed and made him lie down. I said, "Allan, stay put for the next two hours. Drink as much Gatorade as possible. Do you have any chest pain or shortness of breath?"

He shook his head no.

"Don't get up until you feel back to normal. Do everything slowly, okay?" He said, "Okay."

"No more tennis when it is 90°."

Allan recovered completely from his bout of dehydration and hypotension. His driver took him the next day to his office in Westchester. I called Max later in the week, and she said he was doing well. "He is back to normal."

I said, "He still thinks he is Superman and can do anything he wants, whenever he wants. That is all good psychologically, but physiologically he needs some boundaries. Like no tennis when it is over 80°, no skiing without a pro, and no downhill racing with your daughter. I am thrilled he is doing so well physically, but keep an eye on him. Think age-appropriate activity."

Except for a couple of family dinners in Aspen and Southampton, I did not see Maxine or Allan much over the next two years due to my busy operating schedule and family life. Then suddenly Max called me at home one midweek at 9:00 p.m. "Allan is not right . . . he has a cold, but he went to the office all day. He saw an ENT doctor in the city on the way home. The doctor gave him some medication in his office. He was fine during dinner, but now he cannot talk. He is losing his balance and can barely walk."

I answered, "I am on my way."

At age 87, Allan was at the age where patients with cardiovascular disease can often have strokes. This sounded like it could be a possible stroke or a reaction to the medication he took earlier in the day. Either way, he needed immediate attention. Living only three blocks away, I was in the apartment in minutes. Allan was sitting in a chair and was surprised to see me. He couldn't speak intelligibly, he was slurring his words, and he could not stand. His pulse was strong. I said to Max, "He could be having a stroke, or it is a reaction to the medication he took earlier . . . I don't think it is a cardiac problem. Can your driver take us? I will take him to the hospital emergency room. He needs a CT scan of his head and a neurological workup. I can expedite the process in the ER. Ask the doorman to help me get him downstairs to the car. Can you also call the ENT doctor he saw today and find out what medication he gave Allan? Keep your cell phone on, and I will keep you posted."

The emergency room was flooded with patients, but the nurse at the front desk had worked in the Cardiac ICU with me and immediately found Allan a cubicle. The ER attending, who I did not know, came over immediately, and I gave a comprehensive narrative of Allan's medical past. A nurse pulled up Allan's medical hospital record on the computer, and the ER attending said, "It is rare that patients travel with their heart surgeon. We will draw bloods, check toxicology titers, and do a complete workup. I agree with getting a CT scan, and I will have our neurologist look at him . . . have a seat."

Allan was hemodynamically stable, so I knew we were in for a long wait. If the CT scan showed a neuro-deficit (a stroke), he would be admitted to the neurology service. If it didn't, Allan would need to sit in the ER until his neuro status cleared, or until a hospital bed was located. I knew the hospital was very full. On the fourth floor, the cardiac floor, there would be no beds unless someone died. Allan was semi-asleep on his stretcher, and I told the nurse I was going upstairs to look for a bed. I gave her my cell number and said, "Call me if a problem comes up. I will be on the fourth floor."

I ran up the stairs to our ICU. The head nurse said, "No beds." I ran to our step-down unit, "No beds." I tried the next floor, "No beds." I went to the CCU, the last possibility, and the head nurse who I knew well, said, "We have one room, but we are bringing in a patient who is unstable and needs to come to the unit tonight. That will be about 1:00 a.m. Once she is stable and leaves, the bed will open up. Bed control can help clean the room for you, and you can get your patient in there between 2:00 and 3:00 a.m. Would that work?"

I answered, "You are wonderful, thank you very much!"

I ran back to the emergency room just as Allan was wheeled into the CT scanner. He was still groggy, but his vital signs and blood tests were all normal. I called Max at home and asked, "What did you learn from the ENT doctor?"

She said, "He has not returned my calls, so I left a message with his service. How is Allan?"

I replied, "Unchanged. He is going into the scanner now, and I will call you when we get a reading." I ran back upstairs and confirmed with the charge nurse that Allan would get the bed when it opened up. I offered to help clean the room because I was creating work for the nurses that they didn't normally do at 2:00 a.m. She said, "We have it under control. You have other things to do."

I said, "Thank you very much. I owe you big time."

When I got back to the ER, the neuroradiologist had Allan's scan in his hand. "There is no bleeding, no evidence of trauma, no abnormality. It is normal. His mental confusion was caused by the medication he took or lack of sleep or both. We recommend watching him until his head clears here in the ER or in-house if you can find a bed." I said, "Thank you very much . . . I will inform his wife. I am working on a bed."

I called Max and gave her the good news. I said, "I am getting him a bed and expect him to be moved up by 2:00 a.m. He is now asleep, and I expect him to sleep all night and be much better in the morning. My office is just down the hall, so I will keep an eye on him and call you after morning rounds."

At 2:00 a.m., Allan was in his newly cleaned private room. His EKG monitor showed a normal sinus rhythm, and he had normal vital signs. I went to my office down the hall, pulled out my pillow and blanket, and slept on my couch. At 8:00 a.m., on my morning rounds, Allan was still asleep. At 10:00 a.m., he was awake and eating breakfast. He said he "felt fine" and asked me a series of questions about what had happened. After a short explanation, I texted Max, "The big dog is awake and barking. He looks great, his head is back to normal, and he is ready to come home. Send the driver."

BLUE-EYED GIRL

When Lara Chester came into my office with her parents, she wouldn't look at me. She sat in her chair with folded hands, her head tilted forward, eyes looking downward. She had Down's syndrome, and like most Down's patients, she appeared less than half her stated age. Her chart said she was thirty years old, and she had undergone open-heart surgery in another state hospital as an infant for an AV canal defect. She had done well until five years ago when she required a pacemaker for a slow heart rate. She was now having shortness of breath and could only walk a few steps before she had to rest. She could no longer work at the coffee shop where she had been taught to keep the customers' coffee cups full. She normally worked four hours a day, five days a week, and she loved her job. She spent the rest of her day, her mother said, at her group home with five other special needs adults.

Down's syndrome is a chromosomal abnormality associated with intellectual disability, small stature, a characteristic facial appearance, and generalized muscle weakness. Also known as Trisomy 21, it is often associated with valvular heart defects that require urgent surgery in the first years of life. As an infant, her valve lesion had been repaired, but now that repair had calcified and broken down, and her mitral valve was leaking badly. She needed a new valve, and her cardiologist had asked me to see her and plan the surgery. He said, "She has the mentality of a seven-year-old, and the concept of repeat surgery is very frightening to her and her family. Both parents are knowledgeable, and she has three older brothers that help look after her. They are also very protective of her."

I said, "Lara, I want you to meet Pam, my nurse practitioner. She is very nice, and while I talk to your parents, she will show you our hospital. It is a really nice hospital, and I want you to meet the nurses who will be taking care of you, okay? Pam will be your 'special friend' while you are here." I picked up the phone and said, "Pam, can you come in please and show Lara the ICU and the step-down unit?"

When Pam came in, Lara immediately stood up and seemed happy to follow her out of the office. Pam had worked with other Down's patients and knew how to make the hospital less intimidating.

After Lara left, I said to her parents, "Re-operations are always more complicated and higher risk than first-time procedures. There is scar tissue around the heart that makes visibility difficult. Our worst complication in heart surgery is neurological injury, and that risk is 1–2%. There is a 5% risk of bleeding, which would require a repeat visit to the operating room. At Lara's catheterization procedure that Dr. Victor did last month, her coronary arteries looked normal, and her heart muscle was strong. This is good. I think her overall chance of coming through well is 90–95%. The valve we plan to insert will be either made of metal or be a biological valve from a pig. Both have advantages and disadvantages. The metal valve lasts longer, but it would require life-long anticoagulation. Both Dr. Victor and I think that anticoagulants for Lara would be difficult to regulate, so we favor the porcine prosthesis. Do you have any questions so far?" Mr. and Mrs. Chester looked at each other and shook their heads.

I said, "From a timing perspective, this is not an emergency operation. We normally book two weeks in advance. She would be admitted the day prior to the surgery and probably have a week-long stay in the hospital. You think about everything I have said, and call me if questions come up. I am usually scrubbed during the day, but I will call you back in the evening. If you decide to go ahead with the surgery, call Pam or my assistant and set a date.

The next day, they called the office and scheduled surgery for fourteen days later.

When Lara came in for the surgery, she was accompanied by both parents and her three older brothers. I told Pam to greet the family when they arrived and to make them comfortable. The surgery was early the next morning, so I stopped by Lara's room before heading home. As I entered the room, Lara dropped her head and kept her eyes down. I said a quick "Hello" to the family, answered their questions, and headed home.

The operation went surprisingly well. It took two hours to dissect out the scar tissue beneath the sternum and around the heart. I had no trouble going on bypass and arresting the heart. I cut out the old calcified valve and sewed in a new porcine prosthesis. I was very careful to remove all the calcium fragments from the left atrium that could cause a post-op stroke. She weaned off the bypass machine, and the heart muscle remained strong. I gave protamine to reverse the heparin. I closed the chest with eight steel wires, and four and a half hours after the skin incision, we wheeled Lara into the ICU.

I told the nurse taking care of her, "No problems ... I don't want to extubate her tonight. Wait until tomorrow morning." I walked into the family waiting room and said, "She did as well as I hoped. No problems so far. The new valve is working well. You can go in and see her in about one hour. She will be asleep. Once you see her, you are welcome to stay in the hospital, but I recommend you go home. There is nothing you can do for her here. She will not wake up until the morning. If there are any problems during the night, I will call you. I am expecting her to do well."

My discussion with the family was as positive as I could be. I never say, "Everything is perfect, there will be no problems" because surprises do come up. In reality, I am never happy until the patient goes home, and then I still worry. Heart surgery is very invasive, and there is no such thing as a perfect procedure, or a post-op course without challenges and difficulties.

I did a coronary artery bypass operation in the afternoon and left the hospital at 9:00 p.m. On the way out, I stopped by the ICU and checked on Lara. The ICU attending, Chris Adams, one of our best intensivists, said, "She is doing fine, almost no bleeding . . . go get some sleep."

I lived a mile from the hospital, and I always enjoyed my twenty-five-minute walk home in the dark. It is often my only exercise. My family was out of town, so I ate some cereal and went to bed.

At midnight the phone rang, and my beeper went off simultaneously. Not a good sign. Chris Adams was breathless and speaking rapidly. "Her pacemaker suddenly stopped working . . . the temporary wire only works intermittently. Ben is pumping on her chest and is getting a pressure of 80. We called a code."

I said, "Chris, I am ten minutes away; ask the nurses to set up a sternotomy tray at the bedside. Call the OR desk and tell them to get an operating room ready. Call cardiac anesthesia to come in. Have the pump set up, and ask the OR to call the perfusion team. And Chris, lastly, get an emergency electrophysiology consult. Tell them we will probably need a new permanent pacemaker tonight."

I sleep in scrubs, so I put on my tennis shoes and ran down eighteen flights of stairs, as the elevator was slow that night. On the street, I got a cab immediately and was in the hospital in eight minutes. I quickly put on new scrubs and slipped into my OR clogs.

Lara's room in the ICU was crowded with doctors and nurses, all trying to help. The in-house cardiac surgery fellow, Ben Cousins, was steadily pumping on her chest and generating a blood pressure of 80-90mmHg systolic. There was no obvious EKG activity on the monitor. I said, "Ben, you and I will open her chest and put in new temporary wires. We will then get her down to the OR, and we may need to go on pump. She will need a new permanent pacer. The electrophysiology team is on the way to the hospital. We will also do a TEE (transesophageal echocardiogram) to check her valve function."

I put on sterile gloves and positioned myself on the right side of Lara's bed. I painted the chest with fresh beta-dine and draped sterile blue towels around the chest incision. I told Ben to stop pumping, and I rapidly reopened her skin incision. I removed her sternal wires and reopened the chest. Reaching inside, I started massaging the ventricle directly, and I could easily keep her pressure over 100mmHg systolic. There was no blood around the heart and no evidence of cardiac tamponade.

I said, "Ben, while I massage the heart, put two pacing wires on the right ventricle. Hook them to the pacemaker, and see if she captures. I do not see any electrical activity from her permanent leads. Pace her heart at 90 beats per minute."

Fortunately, the heart started pumping immediately with the temporary wires, and I thought it would be safe to transfer Lara downstairs to the OR.

Moving to the OR one floor down with an open chest was always a production. An anesthesia attending, or fellow, had to hand-ventilate the patient. It took three or four residents or nurses to help move the bed. We needed to monitor the EKG and the blood pressure the whole way. I liked to keep my eye on the heart. With an open chest I could accurately observe the heart's activity every second. Luckily, her transfer was uneventful.

In the OR, we carefully lifted Lara onto the table. I personally re-prepped her chest with betadine and put on a new set of sterile drapes. The temporary pacing wires were working well, and her blood pressure was stable. I asked, "Ben, was her pressure ever less than 80mmHg for a pro- longed period of time?" When he answered no, I said to the circulating nurse, "Please ask Chris Adams to stop by the OR so I can talk to him."

I turned to the cardiac anesthesiologist and asked, "Can you pass a TEE probe and look at the LV function and the prosthetic valve? I want to make sure they are okay." He replied, "I think the valve is adequate because the pressure is very stable, but I will take a look."

Chris came into the room, and I said, "Is EP on the way? Something has happened to her permanent pacer, and we need new leads and a new unit. It is five years old. I think the valve is okay, but we will make sure with the TEE probe."

Chris responded, "Dave Lyall from EP is getting changed in the locker room." I asked, "Have you spoken to the family?" He shook his head no. "Could you call them and say the pacemaker malfunctioned and we are putting in a new one? So far, the valve looks fine. I will call them as soon as we come out. Thank you."

When I saw the EP cardiologist at the scrub sink, I made an incision below Lara's left clavicle at the site of her permanent pacing unit. I dissected the battery unit from the surrounding scar tissue.

Dave entered the room, and I said, "Thank you for coming in at this late hour. I know Chris told you the story. If you can give her a new pacing unit, we will be forever grateful."

Sometimes removing old pacing leads can be difficult, but both the ventricular and atrial lead came out easily. Dave replaced both with new screw-in leads that had excellent thresholds. He had brought in a selection of pacemakers, and he was able to replace Lara's old pacemaker with a new unit that was half the size of the old pacer. When he closed the incision, I could barely see the traditional bulge below the left clavicle. The whole procedure lasted only thirty minutes. It was now good to go. "Dave, thank you very much!"

The transesophageal echo demonstrated that the mitral valve was working perfectly, and the left ventricle muscle had not been injured during the night's events. We were also good to go, and Ben and I rapidly closed Lara's chest. There was no significant bleeding, and we transferred Lara upstairs and delivered her back to the ICU nurses at 3:00 a.m.

I thanked Ben Cousins and all the nurses for the excellent help. I went to my office and called Lara's father and mother. "Lara is doing well . . . we put in a new permanent pacemaker and new pacing leads. She looks good, and I will stay in the hospital for the rest of the night. I am not expecting any further problems. Pam or I will call you tomorrow morning. I wouldn't come to the hospital until after 1:00 p.m. She is sleeping quietly now and will not wake up until the afternoon."

At 1:00 p.m. the next day when Lara's parents and brothers came in, she was extubated and talking. She was completely oblivious to the events of the previous night. Her subsequent post-op course was uncomplicated. She loved having Pam visit and walk with her in the hallways, but she continued to duck her head and look down whenever I came into her room. Despite her shyness, I was thrilled with her overall progress, and she was discharged home on post-op day seven.

Five years later at Christmas time, we received a holiday card from the family. The message read:

Dr. Krieger and Pam,

Lara is doing great, back working in the coffee shop. Thank you and your staff,

Merry Christmas!
The Chester Family

Inside the card there was a picture of Lara looking directly at the camera. She had big blue eyes and a wide-open smile.

BACK FROM THE DEAD

Eileen Cunningham was a loyal referral source. She had completed cardiology residency at a time when many women were pushed out of the male-dominated profession. She stayed on the attending staff for several years, and we became friends. As a young female attending, few internists or other cardiologists referred patients to her, so I made it my practice to send her all my cardiac caths and consults. After ten years in the city, she decided to open a new practice out of the city. Despite the existence of excellent local surgical options, she sent all her surgical patients to me, back in the city. I appreciated her loyalty.

One day she called and said, "I have an interesting patient for you . . . he's a biker . . . he doesn't own a car, and he rides into the city every day on a Harley Davidson motorcycle. He looks and dresses like a Hell's Angel . . . lots of tattoos . . . a real tough guy. As a child he was operated on for congenital heart issue . . . thirty years later he was a re-op and had a pig valve replacement. Now he is fifty-five, and the valve is leaking big time . . . he needs a new aortic valve. Can you see him?"

I said, "Send him in, we'll take good care of him."

I was expecting a thickly bearded Hell's Angel-looking biker type, so I was pleasantly surprised when a good-looking middle-aged man with long hair, blue jeans, and leather boots and jacket came into my office. We shook hands in a standard fashion, and I said, "Well, where is the bike?"

He smiled, "It is between two parked cars outside on the street. It is easy to park, and it is the best way to get around in the city. I work in the theater district . . . I'm a driver for actors . . . I chauffeur them around the city when they are filming or in plays. And sometimes when they are filming a movie scene, they stick me in the background. I go from driver to actor!"

We talked about his heart. He knew he needed a new valve. He was getting short of breath at work, and he had swelling in his ankles at the end of each day. "By the time I get home, I have trouble pulling off my boots."

I told him we would admit him to the hospital for several days of testing. This would include a heart catheterization. "We need to look at your coronary arteries and assess the strengths of the heart muscle. If all goes well, we will operate the next day. This will be your third heart operation. There will be scar tissue all around your heart. The operative risk is at least 10%. Our worst complication is a stroke, and that risk is 1–2%. You will be in the hospital seven to ten days post-op, and tell your employers you will not be back for at least six weeks. Can the studios get along without you for that long?"

He grinned, "Not only can they get along without me, they could forget me completely in six weeks!"

I was starting to like this Biker. He wasn't too full of himself. "We will get you back to work as soon as possible. You pick a date and call my secretary. We will take care of the rest."

At catheterization, his aortic valve was leaking badly. His pulmonary pressure was twice normal, and the pulmonary artery was significantly enlarged. The coronary arteries were clean; no bypasses were required. I told his brother, his only family member, that the operation would take five to six hours, twice the normal time. "This is his third operation, and I expect to find thick scar tissue stuck all around the heart."

The next day my suspicion about scar tissue was confirmed. At one of his previous operations, the right pericardium, the sack that encases and protects the heart, had been completely resected. His right lung was plastered over the right ventricle, the pulmonary artery, and the aorta. It took over three hours to dissect out the heart for a safe cannulation. Once cannulated and on bypass, the anesthesiologist turned off the ventilator, and I freed up the right heart structures. I gave up completely on the idea of dissecting out the left heart. To compensate, I would give extra cardioplegia to protect the left heart muscle. I wanted to completely free up the aorta for my cross clamp, but it was stuck to the pulmonary artery. I therefore divided the innominate vein, which was twice normal size. This allowed me to clamp the aorta safely two centimeters above the usual location.

We were now ready to do the "real" operation. I clamped the aortic root and injected cardioplegia to stop the heart. The heart-lung machine was providing blood flow and oxygen to the brain and other organs. I cut out the old prosthetic valve and sewed in a new porcine valve that would hopefully last another twenty years. This is usually the most difficult part of the surgery, but in this case, it would be the most straight-forward part of the whole operation. I closed the incision in the aorta and told the perfusionist to "start warming." It would take an hour to warm him enough so that the heart could take over its normal responsibility of pumping blood to all parts of the body.

When the rectal temperature warmed to 36°C, we weaned the patient off bypass. Now we could assess the new valve function and evaluate the remaining strength of the left ventricle. Both looked good. I said, "Give the protamine first, and the fresh frozen plasma and platelets second." I expected significant bleeding . . . he was a re-op, and the factors from the blood bank would help promote clot formation.

Once the protamine that reverses the effects of the heparin is in, I usually scrub out of the operation. The senior cardiovascular fellow, who would complete his training in three months, would switch to the left side of the table. A surgical physician assistant (PA) would replace him on the right. Normally they would cauterize the bleeding sites, rewire the sternum, and close the subcutaneous tissue and skin.

But not this time. This case was different. This case was not straightforward, and I was worried about the probability of bleeding post-op. I told the cardiovascular fellow, Brad Davis, that I would stay scrubbed until the chest was closed. "With all this scar tissue, bleeding will be a problem . . . I want you to double ligate the innominate vein that we divided at the beginning of the case." I re-clamped the vessels and had Brad tie a 2-0 silk suture for a backup ligature. I over-sewed all the cannulation sites. I put a chest tube in the right pleural space and a large drain above the heart.

I closed the sternum and then scrubbed out. The patient looked dry, and I felt good about the overall operation. The anesthesiologist assured me the new valve and the left ventricle looked "perfect" on the transesophageal echo.

I stayed in the operating room, wrote my notes, and watched the monitors until Brad and the OR staff transferred the sleeping patient on the ICU bed. He was wheeled to the surgical ICU where a gang of ICU nurses would supervise his care. The patient was very stable during this transfer, and I returned to my office pleased that our operation, although long and difficult, had gone well. I was very optimistic for the future of our Biker, Chauffeur, Actor.

Ten minutes later, I was at my office desk with the patient's brother on the phone. "He is doing great . . . it was a difficult operation, but I expect him to make a complete recovery." I had just hung up the phone when my secretary, Jessica, rushed into my office. "There is an emergency call on the other line." I picked up the phone and heard our new faculty member say, "Boss, I'm so sorry to tell you but he's dead . . . I was walking into the unit when they called a code . . . it was your patient from today. I ran in, and we opened his chest. There was a lot of blood . . . he bled out, and we couldn't get him back. I am so sorry to tell you, but he is gone."

I dropped the phone and started sprinting down the corridor to the ICU. How could our patient be "dead"? I had just left him and he was "just fine." He didn't have time to die. Not this fast. I tore open the ICU doors and ran to the bedside. Brad and the new attending stood with their heads hanging down, like the world had come to an end. Even the ICU staff looked morose.

"What the hell happened? He cannot be dead this fast . . . get me some gloves. Brad, run downstairs and tell the OR nurses we are coming back . . . get a pump set up . . . we are going to be there in five minutes . . . we are not letting him die like this."

I looked in the chest cavity, which was full of dark purple blood. This was venous blood, not arterial blood. His heart had stopped beating, but it had not fibrillated like most ICU arrest . . . it was empty and had just stopped beating. I grabbed it with both hands and squeezed it hard, and I saw a small pressure blip on the arterial line monitor.

I yelled, "Pump Ringer's Lactate and all the blood you have into his IV lines. He has bled out . . . give him Ringer's or saline, or anything. I will create the pressure. Give him 4mg of Levophed and 1 gram of Solumedrol, STAT. Give 2mg of Epinephrine and 2 amps of bicarb. Get more blood from the blood bank . . . it can be type-specific . . . and be sure he is hand-ventilated with 100% O$_2$. Start getting him ready to move."

ICU nurses and resident staff were running in all directions. All the time I was talking, I was thinking, *where is the blood coming from?* Venous blood had to originate from the right side of the heart, like our cannulation site, but through the bloody mess I could see the cannulation site, and it wasn't bleeding. Suddenly a lightbulb went on in my head, and I knew what had happened. Brad's tie on the innominate vein must have slipped off, and the vein had retracted and was not visible. Only a big venous structure could cause this much blood loss.

I yelled, "Sponge stick," and the ICU head nurse knew exactly what I wanted. She handed me a 4" x 4" gauze pad on a large Kelly clamp. I stopped massaging the heart long enough to stick the make-do sponge stick into the area beneath the right sternum where the innominate vein would most likely be. Immediately, the bleeding stopped.

Brad had returned, and I said, "Brad, climb up on the bed and hold the sponge stick in the area where it is bleeding. Press hard and do not let go. That is the bleeding site. This is your only job."

We had lost twenty seconds during this interaction, and I returned to massaging the flaccid left ventricle. I knew there had to be some blood in the heart because I was generating a pressure of 50mmHg with each compression. At that moment, for the first time, I knew we had a real chance of saving this guy.

I told the charge nurse, "Call the OR and tell them we are on our way down. Tell them we are going 'back on bypass' and to have the pump team ready for us."

There were at least ten doctors, nurses, and ICU staff in the room, all trying to help. I said, "Let's get ready to move. Someone get the elevator. Brad, you ride on the bed, and I will straddle the patient and keep massaging the heart. I want an anesthesia attending to hand-bag the patient. Is everyone ready? Let's move out."

I am sure we looked like a strange sight headed back to the OR. Nurses were pumping blood into the transfusion lines on both sides of the bed. Two anesthesiologists were hand-bagging the patient and guiding the bed. Brad and I rode on top with our hands in the open chest. There was blood all over the sheets, and it was dripping on the floor. We were leaving a blood trail all the way to the OR. We looked like a mess, but I knew we were making progress.

I was now generating a pressure of 60–70mmHg systolic with my cardiac massage. Brad had the bleeding under control, and I actually felt good. I was confident and determined. We were going to save this guy.

A whole new team of doctors, nurses, and technicians ushered us back into the OR. They helped us transfer the patient onto the operating table where we washed and cleaned his wound as much as possible. Brad and I held our positions on the open chest as we prepped and draped the patient. I asked an OR tech to take Brad's job, and he took mine. I quickly put on my headlight and loops. I scrubbed and put on a sterile gown. Brad then did the same. We draped the patient, and we brought the lines from a new heart-lung machine. Brad put new purse strings in the aorta and right atrium. He took over the cardiac massage, and we heparinized the patient. I placed an arterial cannula in the aorta and a second larger cannula in the right atrium.

"Go on bypass."

As the bypass machine spun into motion, the tension in the room and the pressure on the operating team palpably diminished. We could now catch our breath and take our time. We could let the heart recover from the trauma of the last thirty minutes. The heart-lung machine took over the work of the patient's own heart and lungs and provided enough blood pressure to perfuse the brain and other critical organs. Our patient's heart and lungs were on a temporary vacation.

Our first task was to over-sew the culprit innominate vein. We had double ligated it at the first operation, but the double suture had somehow come off and was nowhere to be seen. I kicked myself as I was hoping not to tear the vessel, but with this particular patient, I needed to tie down even harder. There is always a fine balance to strike when sewing vessels . . . not too tight, not too loose. But this time I sewed the vein closed with 4-0 Prolene, and I tied the knot off.

With the bleeding under control, we examined all our suture lines in the aorta and on the heart chambers. All looked good. We irrigated the chest cavity and pleural spaces with five liters of warm saline. This helped warm the patient, and it diluted any bacteria that might have entered the operating field. The heart, warm and well perfused, started beating spontaneously in a regular rhythm.

I put fresh tubes into both lungs and two drainage tubes in the mediastinal space. I replaced the pacing wires on the right atrium and ventricle so we could control the heart rhythm. The anesthesia team was monitoring the patient's blood gasses and electrolytes. They had transfused eight units of concentrated red cells to restore the patient's blood volume.

The bypass machine was allowing the heart to recover from the insult of the cardiac arrest. When the heart-lung machine was slowed down, I could see the heart contracting in an almost normal fashion. To be safe, I placed an intra-aortic balloon pump in the femoral artery. This cardiac assist device would do some of the work of the left ventricle and help rest the heart.

When the anesthesia team had warmed the patient to 37°C, I said, "Even though he is looking good, let's keep him hypothermic for the next forty-eight hours. This should help protect his brain. I am no longer worried about bleeding."

After only one hour on bypass, we were able to wean off the heart-lung machine. The transesophageal echo miraculously demonstrated normal ventricular function, and the new valve was working well.

When there was no evidence of further bleeding, we removed the cannula and over-sewed the cannulation sites. For the second time that day, we closed the sternal bone with eight steel wires and sutured him to close the subcutaneous tissue and skin.

The patient was completely stable when we transferred him back to the ICU. I was no longer worried about his heart. All bleeding had stopped. The only unanswered question was his head; had his brain tolerated the low blood pressure episode associated with the cardiac arrest?

I knew there was clinical evidence that research patients with low blood pressure secondary to acute heart attacks did better neurologically when treated with forty-eight hours of hypothermia. We would give the hypothermia protocol a test. We cooled our patient to 34° C with a cooling blanket and kept him sedated. Wrapped in the cooling blanket, we could monitor his temperature very accurately. We hoped this would prevent swelling and protect his brain.

Forty-eight hours later we had our answer. After slowly weaning his sedation and warming his core temperature to 37°C, the biker woke up. He moved all his extremities and started breathing without his respirator. His heart rhythm and blood pressure remained completely stable. The neurology service did a thorough neurological exam and found no abnormalities. When he was fully awake, we removed his breathing tube. A repeat echo showed normal cardiac function with no leak around the new valve.

The ICU nursing team was ecstatic about his progress. "In the history of the hospital, we have never seen a patient recover after he was pronounced dead. Never ever. He is 'back from the dead'!"

Despite their enthusiasm, my main concern now was the possibility of wound infection. Opening the chest emergently in the ICU is not done with the same sterile technique used in the operating room. I ordered a seven-day course of intravenous antibiotics.

The next day on rounds, the nurses took me aside and said, "Let us take over his care—we are not going to let him have a wound problem." They rallied around the patient, day and night, and provided the best care possible. Two days later, he was walking in the corridor with a nurse supporting each arm. They made sure he had a quiet sleeping environment. They brought him cookies from home, and after seven days his wound was healing well, and he was walking independently. It was only with their "permission" that I was allowed to transfer him to the step-down unit.

On post-op day eleven, the patient was walking and climbing stairs with "no problems." On post-op day twelve, he asked if he could go home. I said, "You can go home if you promise to stay at your brother's house for two weeks, you cannot ride your bike or go back to work for six weeks, and you have to take it easy."

And I said, "Most importantly, next time you have a role in a movie, you have to let us know."

He gave me a biker/actor handshake and was soon gone.

CONCLUSION AND EMERGING TECHNOLOGY

It has been estimated that more research funding has been raised by federal, state, and private industry to develop new therapeutic tools and medical treatments for cardiovascular patients than any other area in medicine. Despite all this effort, cardiac disease remains the number-one killer in our society.

However, amongst these pessimistic observations, significant progress has been made, and patients with cardiac disease are living longer than ever before. Thousands of patients undergo complex cardiac operations daily that improve the quality of their lives, and dramatically extend their life span.

In this final chapter, I would like to focus on five new exciting areas of technology in cardiovascular care created over the last ten years that will expand the number of patients who can be treated safely and successfully. Much of this technology was not yet imagined even fifteen years ago, and back when I was in medical school, you would have thought this technology was more science fiction than science. Yet, these innovations are already saving hundreds of lives in the United States and around the world.

TAVR

Transcatheter Aortic Valve Replacement is a procedure used to replace a stenotic (or narrowed) aortic valve without requiring open-heart surgery. There is no sternal or chest incision. A catheter is inserted through a small incision in the leg, and a new valve is threaded up the catheter to replace the diseased valve. General anesthesia is not required, the procedure can take less than twenty minutes, and the hospital stay is only two to three days. There is usually immediate relief of symptoms, and heart function is usually improved significantly.

This procedure is ideal for the elderly patient because little or no pain is experienced. The procedure is also ideal for re-operative and high-risk patients, where the heart-lung machine used in conventional surgery would be traumatic and possibly dangerous. Long-term results are excellent.

Robotic Heart Surgery

Robotic heart surgery is a type of minimally invasive surgery done through five small incisions on the side of the chest. There is no sternotomy. A variety of complex cardiac procedures can be done with more precision and control than conventional surgery. Possible operations include coronary artery bypass, mitral valve repairs, cardiac tumor resections, atrial septal defect repairs, maze procedures, septal myomectomies, and tricuspid valve repairs. Robotic surgery is less invasive than conventional surgery with less blood loss, less pain, and less scarring. It also offers a lower infection rate and a shorter recovery period.

There is a significant learning curve for this type of surgery, but this new technology is gaining popularity with patients and surgeons alike.

TEVAR

Thoracic Endovascular Aortic Repair is a new, minimally invasive procedure for the treatment of aneurysms of the thoracic aorta. The aorta that originates at the left ventricle carries blood to all the organs of the body. Unfortunately, it is prone to the formation of aneurysms or areas of dilation and weakness. If this process persists, the aortic wall dilates and may rupture or tear, leading to sudden death.

TEVAR is a minimally invasive technique to repair these aneurysms. It is done through a small incision in the leg with a device called a stent graft. The stent graft is a metal tube covered with fabric that is placed through the groin. It is threaded up the aorta to the area of the aneurysm, where it acts as a scaffold reinforcing the aortic wall and decompressing the aneurysm. It prevents the aneurysm from rupturing, and over time the aneurysm may shrink and close over the stent graft. Patients can often return home after three or four days in the hospital.

ECMO

ECMO stands for Extracorporeal Membrane Oxygenation. The ECMO machine is similar to the heart-lung machine used in open-heart surgery. It is a smaller device that oxygenates and pumps a patient's blood outside the body, and it allows the patient's own heart and lungs to rest and recover. It is generally used until the underlying cardiac or lung condition resolves or improves significantly. It is seldom used over five days, but it is capable of supporting the heart and lungs for over thirty days. It was initially designed to support very ill babies with cardiac or pulmonary insufficiency, but more recently, its application has been expanded to include the hospitalized COVID-19 patient population with pulmonary and cardiac failure. The majority of these patients are intubated and sedated and will require weeks of ICU care.

Most major teaching hospitals have well-defined shock/trauma teams available 24/7 that are capable of initiating ECMO support. Thousands of lives in the United States and around the world during the COVID crisis have been saved with this technology.

VAD

A Ventricular Assist Device (VAD) is an implantable mechanical pump that helps pump blood from the lower chambers of the heart (left and right ventricles) to the rest of the body. It is used temporarily or permanently in people with weakened hearts who suffer from congestive heart failure. When placed in the left ventricle, it is referred to as an LVAD. An RVAD supports the right ventricle. Both devices may be used for either temporary or permanent support. Often LVADs are used for cardiac support while a patient is waiting for a heart transplant. This is referred to as a "bridge to transplant."

If you are not a candidate for a heart transplant but have severe heart failure, a VAD may be implanted as "destination therapy." This includes many very elderly patients. In some cases, after VAD insertion the heart's function can improve spontaneously. This is referred to as a "bridge to recovery," and the VAD can be removed. Regardless of the indication for implementation, most VADs dramatically enhance the patient's quality of life.

GLOSSARY

A

alpha constrictor — drugs that increase blood pressure

ambu bag — device used to provide ventilation

aortic dissection — a tear in the wall of the aorta

arrest — heart stoppage

arrhythmia — abnormal heart rhythm

arterial line — catheter inserted in an artery to measure blood pressure

B

balloon pump — heart support device

betadine — topical disinfectant solution

bicarb — medication used to treat systemic acidosis

blood gas — measurement of blood oxygen and CO2 level

Bovie cautery — electrical device used to stop bleeding

C

CABG — common acronym for Coronary Artery Bypass Graft surgery

cannulate — to insert a tube or catheter into a blood vessel or heart chamber

cardiomyopathy — weakness in heart muscle

cardioversion — electrical shock of heart

cell saver — blood conservation device

central line — venous catheter used for injecting medications

central pressure (CVP) — blood pressure in right atrium

chest tube — tube placed between chest wall and lung

circumflex (CFx) — coronary artery on back of heart

coronary ostia — the opening of a coronary artery into the aorta

CT or CT scan — radiological study of body part

D

defibrillator — device used to shock heart

dialysis — artificial procedure replacing kidney function

Down syndrome (also referred to as Down's syndrome) — congenital chromosomal abnormality

E

ejection fraction (EF) — measurement of heart muscle strength

endocarditis — infection in the heart tissue

EP — electrophysiology, study of heart rhythm

Epinephrine — drug that stimulates heart rate and muscle contraction

F

fibrillation — dangerous abnormal heart rhythm

Foley catheter — catheter inserted into the bladder

H

hand bag — bag that is squeezed to manually ventilates the lungs

Heparin — an anticoagulant used to decrease the clotting ability of blood

HOCM — hypertrophic obstructive cardiomyopathy

hypoxia — low blood oxygen level

I

IABP — intra-aortic balloon pump — heart support device

ICU — intensive care unit

IMA — internal mammary artery — conduit used in bypass operations

innominate vein — vein that empties into the right atrium

inotropes — drugs that stimulate heart function

ischemic — tissue, usually heart muscle, with inadequate blood supply

IV catheter — intravenous catheter

L

left main — most important artery perfusing heart muscle

Levophed — vasoactive drug that increases blood pressure

M

M&M conferences — Morbidity and Mortality weekly conferences

MI — myocardial infarction, heart attack

morphine — narcotic pain medication

O

osteomyelitis — infection in sternal bone

P

perfusionist — technician who manages heart-lung machine

pericardium — fibrous sack that encases the heart

pleural space — anatomic space between the chest wall and lung

protamine — drug that reverses Heparin

pulmonary artery — artery taking blood from heart to lung

pulmonary edema — fluid collection in lung tissue

pump — heart/lung machine used in heart surgery

PVC — premature ventricular contraction

R

Ringer's lactate — electrolyte solution given IV

S

SICU — surgical intensive care unit

sodium bicarbonate — electrolyte solution used in shock

Solu-Medrol — artificial steroid

sternal notch — palpable notch at top of sternum

subclavian artery — branch of aorta inside chest cavity

systemic PH — measurement of blood acid level

T

tamponade — compression on heart by blood or clot

targets — coronary arteries grafted in bypass surgery

TAVR — minimally invasive aortic valve replacement

TEE — Transesophageal Echocardiogram

Teflon felt — artificial material used for surgical support

tidal volume — measure of air in each breath

to shock — electrical charge to heart muscle

to trach — surgical procedure to place tube in trachea

to tube — to place a breathing tube in trachea via mouth

V

ventilator — machine that oxygenates the lungs

volume line — large catheter in systemic vein

X

xiphoid process — palpable cartilage at bottom of sternum

ABOUT THE AUTHOR

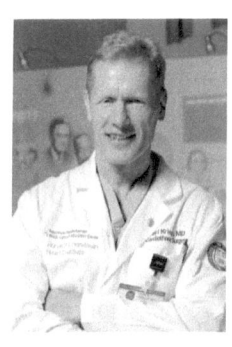

Dr. Karl Hemingway Krieger retired from cardiac surgery in 2022 after a forty-year career in the field of cardio-thoracic medicine. Prior to retiring, he held the positions of the Philip Geier Professor of Cardiothoracic Surgery and Vice Chairman of the Department of Cardiothoracic Surgery at Weill Cornell Medicine. He served as the Director of the Cardiothoracic Surgery Training Program at New York-Presbyterian/Weill Cornell Medical Center. He was also on the Admissions Committee for Weill Cornell Medical College.

After receiving an undergraduate degree from Amherst College, where he studied writing with Tillie Olsen, Dr.

Krieger pursued his medical school education, as well as his surgical internship and residency, at Johns Hopkins. He completed his general surgery and cardiovascular training at NYU Langone Medical Center under the direction of Dr. Frank Cole Spencer. He joined the NYU faculty as a full-time staff surgeon, and Dr. Spencer appointed him the Director of the Cardiovascular Research Laboratory. Dr. Krieger spent over ten years at NYU Langone Medical Center as a full-time staff surgeon.

In 1985, he joined the faculty at Weill Cornell Medicine, under the direction of Dr. O. Wayne Isom, where his responsibilities include teaching medical students, residents, and cardiothoracic fellows, as well as directing a large clinical surgery and research program. He is the author and co-author of over 100 medical articles and abstracts, and he wrote and co-edited the textbook *Blood Conservation in Cardiac Surgery*. Dr. Krieger worked at Weill Cornell for over thirty-five years.

Specializing in high-risk and re-operative surgery, Dr. Krieger is known for his dedication and compassion to his patients. He has expressed, "Each patient should be treated like a member of your family, a mother or a father." Among other awards, Dr. Krieger has received the Maurice R. Greenberg Distinguished Service Award, the Peter Burnett Howe Award, the American Heart Association Distinguished Service Award, and the Stanley V. and Charles B. Travis Award for Academic Excellence. He is most proud of the Physician of the Year award from New York–Presbyterian, for which he was nominated by his nursing staff in 2012.

Dr. Krieger lives in Southampton with his wife, Krista, and has two children, Katherine and Konrad.